PRAISE FOR *Your He...*

"*Your Health Destiny* awakens us from o... ...passive reliance upon pharmaceutical remedies that so often fall short. Selhub's empowering text will transform your perspective, providing the tools to actively and fundamentally change your destiny as it relates to health, disease resistance, and longevity."

> —David Perlmutter, M.D., FACN, author of the *New York Times* bestsellers *Grain Brain: The Surprising Truth About Wheat, Carbs, and Sugar—Your Brain's Silent Killers*

"What you eat, how you move, and what you think are powerful factors that join forces to affect your heart and brain, your strength and immunity. Dr. Eva Selhub knows how each of these manifest in the body and what we can do to support each system. *Your Health Destiny* combines timeless spiritual guidance with the latest medical research on what's best for our bodies and minds, giving you the power to transform your life."

> —Deepak Chopra

"There is a tendency these days to give our health over to our genes and other factors beyond our control. This is a serious mistake. The key insight of *Your Health Destiny* is that our health is not fixed, but can be constructed by the decisions and choices we confront every day. In this important task, let Dr. Eva Selhub be your guide."

> —Larry Dossey, M.D., author of *Reinventing Medicine* and *One Mind*

"Your health is indeed your destiny! You control it with your attitudes, habits and activities. At least 85 percent of all diseases are the results of your choices. Choose wisely from the many great prescriptions in this important book."

> —C. Norman Shealy, M.D., Ph.D., founder and CEO of the National Institute of Holistic Medicine and founding president of the American Holistic Medical Association

"For many, the stresses of modern living can be ever-mounting and more difficult to manage. *Your Health Destiny* presents clear and practical guidance on not only how to face one's stressors but how to overcome them as well. Dr. Eva Selhub skillfully illustrates how to nourish and find balance between one's physical, mental, and spiritual well-being."

—Bardor Tulku Rinpoche, author of *Living in Compassion*

"Dr. Eva has provided an essential guidebook for maintaining optimum health. She goes far beyond the 'fix-it' medical model by providing the reader with an in-depth understanding of how lifestyle choices, environmental influences, and your beliefs can literally change how your DNA expresses itself, as the new science of epigenetics is proving. Dr. Selhub provides education, encouragement, and inspiration that reveal an entirely new way of practicing medicine, yet maintains many elements of ancient wisdom traditions."

—Dr. Steven Farmer, author of *Healing Ancestral Karma, Earth Magic,* and *Sacred Ceremony*

"Dr. Selhub's book gives you the theory, practice, and—most important—the steps to living a full and successful life. She shows you how to take control of your health in a step-by-step manner and develop the method for you to be your own boss. She draws on her enormous experience with patients and her own life's journey to present a guide to change your life. I highly recommend this book to help change behavior and develop the techniques to get the most of your life while defeating stress. All this comes through knowledge and your practicing her simple method of changing your present to brighten your future."

—John J. Ratey, M.D., clinical associate professor of psychiatry at Harvard Medical School and author of *Spark*

EVA SELHUB, M.D.

YOUR
Health
DESTINY

How to Unlock Your Natural Ability
to Overcome Illness, Feel Better,
and Live Longer

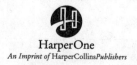

HarperOne
An Imprint of HarperCollins*Publishers*

HarperOne

This book contains advice and information relating to health care. It should be used to supplement rather than replace the advice of your doctor or another trained health professional. If you know or suspect that you have a health problem, it is recommended that you seek your physician's advice before embarking on any medical program or treatment. All efforts have been made to assure the accuracy of the information contained in this book as of the date of publication. The publisher and the author disclaim liability for any medical outcomes that may occur as a result of applying the methods suggested in this book.

HarperCollins books may be purchased for educational, business, or sales promotional use. For information please e-mail the Special Markets Department at SPsales@harpercollins.com.

HarperCollins website: http://www.harpercollins.com

FIRST HARPERCOLLINS PAPERBACK EDITION PUBLISHED IN 2016

Heart Diagram: Copyright © by Nucleus Medical Art, Inc. / Getty Images

Immunity Chart: Copyright © by www.myvmc.com

Designed by Ralph Fowler / rlfdesign

ISBN 978-0-06-232779-6

Library of Congress Cataloging-in-Publication Data

Selhub, Eva M.
    Your health destiny : how to unlock your natural ability to overcome illness, feel better, and live longer / Eva Selhub, M.D. — First edition.
        pages   cm
    ISBN 978-0-06-232778-9 (hardcover)
    1. Mind and body therapies.   2. Mental healing.   3. Health.   I. Title.
RC489.M53S45   2015
613.2—dc23   2014031303

16 17 18 19 20   RRD(H)   10 9 8 7 6 5 4 3 2 1

I dedicate this book to my parents, Jacob and Shirley Selhub,
for beating the medical odds, defying their diagnoses,
and proving to me that it is indeed possible to
change our health destiny for the better.

Contents

Your Health Destiny

Healing is a matter of time, but it is sometimes
also a matter of opportunity.

—HIPPOCRATES

When our body gets sick, we often feel out of control. Worse yet, when we have to go see a doctor, we can feel even more vulnerable, perhaps even helpless. We go because we want to hear that there is a remedy, a cure. We take the prescribed medication, have that expensive test done, or go see yet another specialist. We fearfully await lab results. Even if the results turn out to be normal, the feeling of relief is brief, because in the end, when we again fall prey to sickness, we will go through the same cycle all over again.

It does not have to be this way. We do have control over our health, and we can make choices that can positively influence any health issue, big or small, acute or chronic.

The truth is, we are supposed to get sick; it's the body's way of telling us there's a problem. The belief that there is some kind of absolute or perfect state of health gets us into trouble, because it drives us to desperately accept answers from health-care professionals without also tuning into our body's needs and strengths. When the body gets sick, it's a sign that we are out of balance, and it's not just a time to seek help from our doctors, but also a time to take responsibility and empower ourselves as experts on our own health.

Your body and its processes do not have to be an enigma to you, and it is through understanding that you can find your power to heal and thrive. It is really your choice to do so.

Take Brittany's case. Brittany woke up one morning unable to move her neck. She panicked. She had been in a car accident two years earlier and had sustained an injury to her cervical spine. It had been fine for years. The worst possible scenarios coursed through her mind: "I have a bulging disc. There is nerve damage. I will be paralyzed. I can't afford to be immobilized—not today; I have so much to do and so many commitments to attend to. Damn, I can't work out. God help me, I am in so much pain."

Brittany was thirty-two years old, very active, and healthy, by her own standards. She exercised daily, ate three meals a day, worked as a nurse, took care of her three children, and managed to say yes to every parent committee that the school had. As she lay in her bed in excruciating pain, she wondered how she would manage.

She went to see her primary-care physician, who gave her several prescriptions—a pain medication, a muscle relaxer, and a sleep aid—and a referral to a neurosurgeon for an MRI (magnetic resonance imaging). After leaving the office, Brittany burst into tears and called me, as she had come to see me before to learn how to manage her stress more effectively.

"I don't want to take all these medications," she cried. "I don't want there to be something wrong with me. I have so much to do. I have so many obligations. I am so stressed as it is. I can't move my neck. What if it's something really bad? I don't want surgery."

I didn't interrupt Brittany as she cried and complained. I gave her the space to express her fears without trying to tell her everything would be okay or give her advice, not at the outset. Soon Brittany was able to able to relax into my silence and take some deep breaths with me.

Then I spoke. "What we are doing right now is creating space for your magnificent body to heal. Whatever is going on is fixable. Remember that. You are in control, not me, not the neurosurgeon, and certainly not your pain. Your pain is, however, trying to tell you something, perhaps something more than just that your spine may be out of alignment. It's trying to tell you that your life may be out of alignment too, as what is transpiring within your body often mirrors your experiences in your everyday life. For instance, your pain may be telling you that you have been functioning under stress and duress and that you might want to slow down. It may be telling you that you tend to get overwhelmed and out of balance, because you take on too much responsibility and have a hard time saying no when asked to do something or help someone, at the same time that you are unable to accept help or support from others."

I instructed Brittany to take only the muscle relaxer at night for two or three days, which would help her sleep and also remind the muscles how to relax. I taught her breathing exercises and guided meditations that she could practice regularly that focused on allowing the universe to soothe, love, and guide her. During this rest period, Brittany was also to journal about why she felt so obligated to be so busy and help others so much, even at her own expense, and follow this with a description of her values, virtues, and victories that make her special and the unique person she is.

Within four days, Brittany's pain subsided, so that she was almost back to feeling her usual self, but she had more awareness now. Her rest period had given her the opportunity to reflect and realize that underlying her behaviors and actions was a belief that she wasn't "enough," that she was a failure at really "getting things done, unlike other people," making her want to push harder and do more. She was ready to reprogram this belief into one of knowing she is enough.

And just like that, Brittany went from feeling out of control to being in control of her health. She still planned on meeting with the neurosurgeon and getting the MRI, but now she did not feel that she had to accept whatever he or she said. This experience had shown her that her body, when given the opportunity to do so, had an incredible capacity to heal itself, and when she was guided to listen deeply to the messages her body had to reveal to her, she could learn how to improve the alignment and support not only in her spine, but also in her life.

The good news is, you don't have to wait until you are really sick or in pain to start making different choices. I have treated thousands of patients who have had a myriad of problems—from heart disease to cancer, depression to anxiety—who learned to make better choices that supported and stimulated their body's tremendous natural healing power. Board-certified in internal medicine, I know how to treat most medical ailments, and I understand that when your back hurts, you just want the pain to go away, and you are willing to do or take anything. I also know that when you improve your lifestyle choices, your beliefs, and your emotions and, most important, address how you approach the stress in your life, your need for medications or Western medical intervention subsides or ceases. I will not tell you to stop taking your medication. I will tell you that there are tools and prescriptions available to you that have no side effects and can often get you off your medications or at the very least lower the dosages.

The human body is a living, breathing system. It is in a constant state of flux as it responds to changes in the internal and external environment. When out of balance or facing a challenge, it will let you know through symptoms and illness, so that you can do something about it and actually get better. It is important to listen to and respond to these messages; if you ignore or cover them over, the situation will only get worse.

Modern medicine focuses on getting rid of symptoms and managing body parts, so that you can continue on with your life; it does not address the real core issues of why you are in the state you are in to begin with or the reason the body is reacting the way it is in the first place. Medications like ibuprofen, for instance, are prescribed to treat inflammation, which helps your pain, so that then you can continue doing whatever you normally do. The problem is that inflammation is a natural warning signal for you to do something different, not to keep doing the same thing you've been doing. This is the problem with just treating symptoms! It is when you do not heed the body's whispers that you usually suffer the consequences of its screams.

Choosing to smoke cigarettes or breathe clean air can have a markedly different effect on your lungs. You know that. Choosing which foods you eat, organic versus highly processed and full of chemicals, directly affects your health. You know that too. What you may not know is that the mind has an incredible power to activate the healing capacity of the body. Though our Eastern neighbors have understood this for a long time, modern Western medicine is slowly catching up. Scientific research is showing us that you can even change the way your DNA expresses itself by the choices you make. For example, even if you have a family history of heart disease combined with initial symptoms, the disease can be completely reversed with better lifestyle choices.

The Process of Taking Control

We ultimately do not fully understand why disease occurs. We all have strong cells and weak ones within us. Sometimes our immune system is strong enough to fend off invaders, and other times the system fails. Modern medicine is occupied with figuring out how to kill off cancer cells and viruses, but it would be in our best interest to instead help our immune system get stronger and support our body's natural healing mechanisms.

I have found that when patients choose to see themselves as having enough resources to manage adversity, they are ultimately healthier and more resilient. In contrast, the patients who consider themselves victims of life's circumstances are less likely to handle challenges or trauma effectively or adaptively, and this includes those individuals who hand their health over to experts. They are more likely to succumb to negative emotional, psychological, and physical complaints and thoughts, which, in turn, creates more stress, further weakening the mind and the body. There is little benefit in seeing oneself as a victim, no matter the hardship.

In my practice, patients learn to take charge of their own health destiny by doing the following:

1. Addressing the problem from an allopathic medical perspective: medication, interventions, lab draws, and so on.

2. Supporting the body with appropriate physical exercises and tools, such as nutrition, stretching, adequate sleep, and so on.

3. Working on creating the social infrastructure they need to feel supported enough to heal.

4. Learning about physiology and becoming acquainted with their body's unique signals for help.

5. Releasing and reprogramming deep-seated negative emotions and beliefs.

Based on the latest scientific research and my clinical experiences, this book contains the prescriptions you need to transform your health now and in the future. You will learn how to pay attention to your body's whispers, to understand what these signals mean, and then make the right choices that will bring amazing results to your health, in both the short and long term. You will discover ways to prevent disease from happening or getting worse, and you may find that you can reverse the disease process altogether.

Your Choice to Take Charge

Throughout this book I will guide you through the process of developing the systems your body and mind need to stay strong and vibrant. I will help you develop awareness of the body's anatomy, from the spine to the heart to the mind, and how all parts are connected to make one unit by providing you with the pertinent medical and scientific knowledge. I will also show you how to hone your perception of your physiology and increase your ability to uncover subtle imbalances that may be harming your health. Finally, I will offer you reprogramming tools and active steps that can help you heal your mind, body, and soul in ways that will improve not only your health, but your life as well.

Over the course of my twenty-year career at Harvard Medical School, Beth Israel Deaconess Medical Center, Tufts Medical School, and the Benson-Henry Institute at Massachusetts General Hospital, where I served as medical director and staff physician, I have discovered a fundamental truth: for most people, health, happiness, and strength are a result of the affirmative choices we make despite what life hands us, whether in our genetic makeup, our environment, or the things that happen to us.

If we choose to be happy, we can be.

If we choose to be healthy, we can be.

If we choose to be strong, we can be.

If we choose to change our health destiny, we can.

CHAPTER ONE

The Power to Transform Health

The part can never be well, unless the whole is well.

—PLATO

Like the weather, your health is constantly changing. This fact alone provides you with choice. You have a tremendous ability to influence that change. Simply put, you have the power to transform your mind and improve the functioning of your body. The key to this power lies in your ability to bounce back from illness, manage life's stress efficiently and effectively, and truly believe in the possibility of good.

A meta-analytic review of the effects of optimism on physical health done at the University of Kansas in 2010 found that optimism was a significant predictor of positive physical health outcomes.[1] Laura Kubzansky, an associate professor at the Harvard School of Public Health, has found through her research that optimism can cut the risk of coronary artery disease in half. She says about genes: "They are 40–50 percent heritable, which means you may be born with the genetic predisposition. But this also suggests there is a lot of room to maneuver."[2] In other words, there is wiggle room in the power you have to positively influence your health.

The notion that you have a lot of "wiggle room" with your genes is an empowering fact. The burgeoning science of epigenetics tells us that by changing our environment, from stressful to nurturing, we can affect how a gene's DNA expresses itself. Why is this so important?

Genes and the Environment

The drastic changes in lifestyle and human social habits during the last fifty years has been linked to the rise in such diseases as obesity, diabetes, sleep disorders, depression, and certain types of cancers, disorders associated with disturbances in the circadian rhythm, or the internal timekeeper in each of your cells. This timekeeper, or clock, is connected with your stress response and stress hormones and is associated with "clock genes." These clock genes have a strong impact on many biological functions like memory formation, energy metabolism, and immunity. A recent review in the *Journal of Neuroscience* shows that environmental factors like stress, drug abuse, or poor sleep habits compromise the circadian rhythm, causing the genetic landscape of your "clock genes" to change its shape.[3] For instance, sleep loss causes subsequent changes in these clock genes, which then negatively affects these processes.[4] Have you ever noticed that when you lose sleep, especially for a few days in a row, you have difficulty remembering anything, your metabolism slows down, and you are more prone to catching that nasty bug that is going around? You also likely have experienced the reverse, when a little more sleep goes a long way in improving these symptoms.

Herbert Benson, a physician at Boston's Massachusetts General Hospital, has found that meditation not only improves health outcomes and brain function, but can also positively affect the expression of genes. An analysis revealed that pathways involved in energy metabolism were up-regulated during the relaxation response, or the meditation practice, meaning that metabolism improved. Pathways known to play a prominent role in inflammation, stress, trauma, and cancer were suppressed, meaning there was less inflammation. The expression of genes involved in insulin pathways was also significantly changed for the better, implying better regulation of blood sugar.[5]

These clock genes and the genes examined in Benson's study are intricately connected with the wiring in the brain. The ever-expanding science of neuroplasticity, or the examination of how the brain continues to change and remodel, confirms that, by adjusting the environment in the mind and body through diet, emotional balance, better stress management, more sleep, and more time in nature, it is possible to create positive changes in the brain resulting in improved health and well-being. In other words, by lowering the stress your body is exposed to and by improving your lifestyle habits and behaviors, you can actually change the course of your health for the better; the landscape of your brain and your genes improve.

Stress to your system does not come only in the form of the food you eat or a lack of sleep, but also in the thoughts and beliefs you hold and the negative emotions that can run rampant through your brain. Without addressing the mind, your beliefs and emotions, and the biochemistry and physiology of the body, the behavior and lifestyle changes you need to make simply will not stick.

Your thoughts, emotions, and beliefs, and therefore your perception of yourself and your world, are directly connected to your body's biochemistry and physiology. Research tells us that your beliefs can affect your body's biochemical responses and that you have the power to believe in good and thus feel good.[6] When you expect good, and I mean really believe that a good outcome is possible, your body responds positively. The catch is that you also need to believe in and support your body's strength and natural ability to heal. Expecting your body to be strong without supporting it does not work. You have to choose to change your mind and your attitudes toward health and your life for the good, so that good can also manifest itself in your body.

Are you as excited about this fact as I am? You should be, because it implies the possibility that changing the landscape of your beliefs and thoughts, not just your sleep habits, can offset your clock genes for the better. You actually have an active choice in what thoughts or beliefs you hold at any given moment in life. You can choose to be happy or choose to be miserable. You can choose to look at yourself, your life, and your predicaments from the standpoint of a victim, or you can choose to be a victor in the adventure that is your life.

If this sounds as though I am telling you that all you have to do is "Don't worry, be happy," I am not. It is not that simple. Fear and stress are naturally present in the world and in our bodies, but you have the ability to control your reactions, move beyond your negative emotions, and achieve a greater sense of well-being.

Emotions and Well-Being

Your emotions and your emotional memory are directly connected to physiological responses, both positive and negative. When you face a challenge in your current life, your brain searches its memory bank to see how you have handled such a situation before and what you know about it. It will also try to match your current emotion to one in your data bank of emotional memories. When it does, your brain will respond in kind with automatic assumptions and physiological reactions associated with it. So if for the past five years you have experienced repeated pain, it is unlikely that you will really believe that next month you will be pain free or at least suffer less. You will be more likely to be fearful and apprehensive when thinking about it and throw "Don't worry, be happy" out the window. In other words, stress and fear win out.

You can see for yourself how your emotions affect your physiology:

AWARENESS EXERCISE

Think of a situation that you are stressed about. Perhaps you are angry with someone or something or feel anxious, worried, or upset. Choose a situation in which you feel you have little control over the outcome.

Notice how you feel. Notice how strong the emotion is that you are experiencing. Notice the thoughts that come up for you. Be aware of the sensations you are experiencing in your body, particularly in your chest, jaw, stomach, and the movement of your breath.

Now redirect your focus and think of a situation of awe, love, or laughter. For instance, you might remember how it felt to be looked at by someone who absolutely adores you, when you watched your child walk for the first time, gazed at an incredible sunset, or laughed so hard you couldn't breathe. Try to stay in this experience for a minute or two.

Once you have spent some time with the positive experience, go back to thinking about the stressful situation and notice if you feel or think differently.

You may notice that you do feel differently, in your body. You might also observe that you feel slightly differently, perhaps less charged, about the situation. By changing your emotion, you change your experience of the current problem, and therefore your perception of it, even if only slightly at first.

The key here is that when you change your physiology from stress to balance, you are able to change your emotion and then have access to positive expectation. When you don't make this necessary change, stress, fear, and the ensuing physiology tax your body, your health, and ultimately the strength you actually have to heal. The more pressing problem is that you may not even realize how much stress you are under and how overtaxed your body is.

The Body Whispers Stress Before It Screams in Pain

Most of you probably will admit to having a lot of stress in your life. You also know whether you feel good or not; whether your life is moving smoothly or not; and whether you feel you have or are enough or not. What you may not know is that every time the answer is "not," you are in stress, or more specifically your body is in stress.

Your body lets you know that it is in stress by causing you some kind of discomfort—physical, emotional, mental, or psychological. Experiencing hunger? The body is letting you know it needs food, that you don't have enough fuel. Feeling tired? The body is letting you know it needs rest, that you don't have enough energy. Feeling frustrated? The body is telling you to reassess your situation, because you are not getting your needs met, that you are not, perhaps, feeling validated enough.

The body first communicates subtly, in whispers—a pang in the neck, a tingle in the stomach, a slight feeling of being run down or out of sorts. It speaks to you through emotional symptoms—like overwhelming sadness or experiences of annoyance. It communicates through your own thoughts, whether they are judgmental notions about yourself or worries regarding your future.

Through discomfort of one kind or another—physical, mental, emotional, or psychological—the body lets you know that there is an underlying problem it would like you to address. It has to do it this way; otherwise you would not know when it was time to eat, sleep, or change positions. For instance, if you sat in the same position for ten hours and your body did not make you conscious of some sort of discomfort, you would not move and your muscles would atrophy. Now imagine that your body did register discomfort, but you could not move because you were trapped. The mild discomfort would become outright pain. Your mild irritation might turn into outright panic. Your body is no longer whispering; it is now screaming for help.

When stress accumulates and is not taken care of, the stress response, which uses every system of your body, goes into overdrive, taxing your body and ultimately its fighting power. For example, high levels of chronic stress can deplete your immune system, causing you to be more susceptible to viruses or infections.

Walter Cannon, a Harvard physiologist, coined the term "fight or flight" in the 1930s to describe our inborn defense response to threat or danger. He believed this defense response is meant to ultimately ensure survival.[7] When we face a threat or danger, the release of stress hormones like adrenalin and cortisol into the bloodstream catapults us into a state of readiness, our senses become aroused and hyperalert, our pupils dilate to allow in light, and peripheral vision is blocked to enable us to hone in on what must be done. Our muscles tense to prepare for battle or flight. The liver releases stored sugar into the bloodstream, while the breathing rate becomes faster and the breath more shallow to economize on oxygen consumption. Blood flow is diverted to the brain, heart, large muscles, and lungs to make sure the oxygen gets to the areas that will be used to mount our defenses (as opposed to the digestive tract or reproductive system). These are all great defenses when a tiger is chasing you—not so much when your body wants to rest and heal.

To your brain, it doesn't really matter what stressor you are facing. Endocrinologist Hans Selye, in the 1950s, expanded on Cannon's work and explained that you do not have to be chased by a raging animal for the fight-or-flight response to be triggered; this heightened reaction occurs regardless of whether the challenge at hand is life threatening or not.[8] You could be late for work, preparing for public speaking, or worried about paying your mortgage. To your brain, stress is stress.

What you may want to be clear on is what the definition of stress actually is: any threat or challenge to your state of stability, or homeostasis. This could be a change in your blood-sugar levels or the fact that the temperature outside has dropped twenty degrees.

And when you experience any kind of stress, your brain initiates physiological corrective responses that will bring your body back into a state of stability, which can range from regulating your body temperature to finding shelter, food, or love. In other words, stress is not necessarily "bad," but rather the real reason you are able to maintain and sustain life, or pretty much do anything.

The problem is not so much stress, but the inability to manage it and resume stability. You see, the body is constantly moving in and out of homeostasis. You are comfortable, then you are uncomfortable, then you shift positions, and you are comfortable again. This process is called allostasis, or the ability to achieve stability through change.[9] Not being able to make a change to bring about comfort or stability creates a problem, or an allostatic load.

Let's just say you are exposed to a virus during your very stressful day at work, when you barely have time to eat lunch, let alone manage to eat something that isn't fast food. By the time you get home, you notice you feel more tired and achy than usual, but chalk it up to the stressful day, brew some coffee, and get to working on (and worrying about) your next project. Unbeknownst to you, your stress response is working too, kicking your immune system into action, and the inflammatory products that are flying through your bloodstream are causing you to feel more fatigued.

This is the important part: your immune system has kicked in to fight the infection and create a sense of fatigue to motivate you to rest, so it can work more efficiently and effectively. But you do not rest. You stay up late working on your project. Your immune system works overtime, and the next day you find yourself immobilized with profound fatigue and a high fever.

You see, the whole time you had choice. At any point along the way you could have chosen to listen to your body's symptoms, taken heed, and employed more self-care. Your ability to bounce back from a viral invasion could have been drastically improved, thus altering the destined course of your health. You could have, for example, gone home, rested, perhaps taken an Epsom-salt bath, and eaten some chicken soup, which is loaded with healthy vitamins and minerals that support your immune system, and perhaps you never would have succumbed to the virus.

This is true for every aspect of your life and health. You always have the ability to make empowered choices that enable your body to heal itself, choices that keep your stress levels down and the stress response active only when it is needed to do its work. Being exposed to a virus, for instance, does warrant the activation of the stress response and the immune system. You want the stress response do to its job and help your body get rid of the virus. When the work is done, you also want the stress response to turn itself off, so that your system can get back into its steady state. Adding more stress to the equation with your beliefs, habits, and behaviors is only going to push the response to stay active, become overactive, and maybe even burn out, so that your symptoms lead not just to a passing illness, but a full-blown disease.

You're in control.

Making an Empowered Choice

Having said that, even when you have been diagnosed with a "disease," whether it is cancer or heart disease, you still have the power to make different choices that will keep the stress response more controlled, which prevents the problem from worsening and the symptoms from rearing their ugly heads. You might even discover that the process can be reversed altogether.

Let's say you receive a diagnosis confirming that something is "wrong with you." Perhaps you are told you have "carcinoma in situ," a precancerous condition that often progresses to cancer. How would you react? If you are like most people, you would feel scared, worried, and anxious. Your mind would jump to automatic negative assumptions, and the extent of the negativity would depend on how bad you perceive your diagnosis to be. This negative emotional state stimulates your stress response to varying degrees and for a multitude of reasons, including but not limited to the stress in your life that is already present, the stress of the actual disease process, and stress that comes from fear and apprehension of the unknown.

You don't want to be told that you are not well, whole, or intact. Just knowing there is something wrong with you can get you trapped in a loop of negative thoughts, emotions, and beliefs, which could have negative physiological implications caused by a heightened fight-or-flight response, including increased blood pressure, muscle tension, and inflammation. These physiological changes, in turn, can negatively affect your body's natural ability to heal, your own capability to cope and function, and ultimately your belief that overcoming this diagnosis is possible.

In reality, a diagnosis reflects a pattern of discordance or imbalance in the body that is caused by a variety of factors—genetics and lifestyle behaviors are just two of them. When my patients understand they are not their diagnosis, nor are they prisoners to it, they start the process of breaking free from limiting beliefs and labels, enabling them to open the door to the possibility of a positive outcome. They begin to perceive that their illness or life problem is a challenge that *can* be reckoned with, that other options for an outcome are possible, and that they have a choice about how they handle their situation. They have a choice to expect good. And science does show that positive expectation can confer better health.

Think about it yourself. If you were told you had diabetes, what would it make you think about and how would you feel about it, about your chances of getting better and the idea of now having to take medication? Conversely, what if you were told that your body was showing an imbalance in its ability to process sugar? Would you feel the same or think the same thoughts? I personally would feel more in control when presented with the latter explanation, so I could think of it as just needing to find a way to get my system more balanced. In other words, I am more likely to believe in the possibility of a positive outcome. When a diagnosis is made, you have two choices—feeling scared and powerless or responding with hope and the belief you can change your health destiny.

Which brings me back to the power of expecting good. A diagnosis is not necessarily a bad thing when you have a set of tools that enable you to make healthy life choices and change your beliefs about illness and health. Beliefs are the result of where you choose to put your focus. When you choose to focus on what you can do, not what you can't, you successfully change your beliefs and begin to expect good. When you expect good, your stress response lightens up, and your body's chances of healing improve.

What will *you* choose?

CHAPTER TWO

Choosing Healthy, Choosing Happy

The greatest force in the human body is the natural
drive of the body to heal itself—but that force is not
independent of the belief system. Everything begins with
belief. What we believe is the most powerful option of all.

—NORMAN COUSINS

t is New Year's Eve. You raise your glass of Champagne and toast the
New Year, pledging that *this* is the year that you will finally get in
shape. You plan on actually going to the gym that you have been paying for monthly, eating more vegetables and less fast food, and drinking less caffeine. A month later you find yourself eating nachos and
telling yourself that you will start tomorrow. Your excuse for failing
again? Stress. You are too stressed out, and you need comfort.

Trying to stop old habits that help you manage through the stress
you experience can be as challenging as trying to stop a shiver when
you are cold. Your habits are automated patterns that have been active
for a long time and have therefore become "habituated." If these behav-

iors didn't have a history of helping you feel better, at least in the short term, on a consistent basis, you wouldn't be doing them today. Physiologically, these habits do turn the stress response off, as neurotransmitters like dopamine and serotonin are released and reward systems in your brain are activated, but it is temporary. The stress response rears its ugly head again soon thereafter, either because of your guilt or negative emotion, because the problem you're stressed about still persists, or because the habit itself is unhealthy.

For example, you may have a tendency to overeat foods high in sugar when you feel overwhelmed or stressed. The sugar is not necessarily taking care of whatever you are worried about, but it is causing your serotonin levels to rise and stimulating the dopaminergic reward centers in your brain. The result is that you feel better. Thus the term "comfort food." But the effect is temporary, and you are still overwhelmed by your problems. In addition, your body is also stressed by the excess sugar, the stimulation of insulin, the inflammatory response, and any negative emotions you may be experiencing, like guilt or shame for having just eaten something "bad" or for being unable to maintain the promise you made to give up sweets. Feeling worse, you eat more sweets.

I can use myself as an example. Before I started using my own prescription, I used to ignore my feelings of anxiety or inadequacy. I chose to pay less attention to my body and what I could not control and more to the things that gave me instant gratification and feedback, so that I could keep working. I poured myself into my work, into writing, spending time on the Internet, and eating delicious, yet fattening foods. I made myself so busy that I had little time or energy for other things, especially for exercise. I tried to boost my energy with more comfort foods and caffeine and then felt guilty about my actions. To override the guilt, the "What the Heck Effect" would kick in. You know the effect. You say to yourself, "I cheated and screwed up anyway. What the heck! I might as well screw up the rest of the day." And so I ate my favorite baked or fried foods, only to find myself feeling more fatigued, out of sorts, and of course fat. And the cycle raged on until I decided to actually learn how to control my stress response.

What do I mean by controlling the stress response? Let's use the simple example of sitting in a stressful meeting with your boss, while also desperately needing to use the restroom. You are anxious about how your boss perceives you and how he might criticize you and you are also physically stressed because your bladder is about to burst. You can barely concentrate, let alone think clearly, your heart is racing, your stomach hurts, you feel as though you can't breathe, and your neck muscles are tight.

You finally get a break and use the restroom. Relief at last. You can at least focus and breathe now, but you still don't want to go back into the meeting because your fears of inadequacy or of being evaluated poorly are still high. The pit of your stomach hurts, and your shoulders are still scrunched up to your ears.

But then imagine that during your break you decide instead to do a quick relaxation exercise, work on some affirmations that help you let go of your feelings of inadequacy, and remind yourself of everything you have accomplished during the past year. In other words, you manage to quiet your stress response by addressing physical, emotional, and cognitive components of it through relaxation, affirmation, and reframing your thoughts to more positive ones. You actually find yourself feeling not only physically relieved, but also more empowered as you go back into the meeting.

When the stress response is turned off, reward systems in your brain are activated, feel-good chemicals are released into circulation, and you are able to think more clearly, feel more relaxed, and be less anxious. But if you only address one component and not the underlying way you perceive and react to stress in general, this relief is temporary at best.

You want to be able to address every aspect of stress that you can in order to better control your response to it, as Jenna did. Jenna was forty-nine when she came to see me, complaining of insomnia that had been worsening over a twelve-year period. Recently, she had developed panic attacks as well. She complained that her doctors had put her on multiple medications for insomnia, anxiety, and depression, but these were not helping. The only remedy that worked was wine—two glasses a night to be specific.

Jenna told me that her childhood had been very difficult, because her mother was in and out of mental institutions regularly, leaving Jenna to take care of herself. With little money, provisions, or support, she often felt alone and overwhelmed. In high school, she found herself finally being accepted by a group of kids and remembered those years fondly. It was then that she discovered that alcohol soothed her nerves.

Fast-forward to adulthood. Jenna worked as a successful bank manager and was married with three grown children. She was surrounded by people who respected and adored her, yet she admitted she still harbored feelings of low self-esteem and shame. She believed she could never be "enough" for anyone and never really belong anywhere. She put extra pressure on herself to meet every deadline, take care of every complaint her children had, and please her husband. Yet she felt like a failure at everything. She worried that if she did not work hard at work or in her marriage, she would find herself alone and destitute again.

Jenna's insomnia and anxiety were certainly problematic. But they were also symptoms of an overactivated stress response resulting from multiple stressors, including the hassles of everyday life, her underlying beliefs that she would never be good enough or belong, and her fear of not having enough to survive, despite having an overflowing bank account.

For Jenna, the first step toward feeling better was to understand the underlying cause of her stress, what stress really meant for her, and its different facets, including uncovering her underlying fears of not being loved or supported. In addition to learning new coping strategies and implementing lifestyle changes, Jenna also had to discover the ways in which her body whispered when the triggers for feeling "not enough" were activated and use healthier tools to alter the belief to one of being enough.

By addressing Jenna's needs to feel loved, valued, supported, and relevant, it was possible to quiet her stress response, so that she could address the real challenges in her life with a clear mind and a relaxed body. Within three months, Jenna's sleep improved and her anxiety attacks ceased, never to appear again, and she no longer needed to self-medicate with wine.

Like Jenna, many of us have underlying fears and assumptions that drive our behaviors or habits. Most of them developed early in life. Over the course of our lifetime, as one memory built upon another, a belief system formed, and we developed our own conclusions regarding how we see ourselves, others, and the world around us. Some of our beliefs hold positive expectations that our future needs will be met. Other beliefs, based on more hurtful experiences, take a more negative stance, holding negative expectations that we may never be or have enough and that the world or people can't be trusted to help us.

For instance, if in your past your family always had enough money and money was never an issue, you will likely believe today that you will always have enough money if you should need it. In contrast, if you grew up in a home where food and clothing were always in short supply or sometimes unavailable, your experience will be that of not having enough money. As an adult now, even though you have a stable income, you still may wonder, "What if I won't be provided for? What if I don't have enough money? What if I can't pay my rent?" So you worry daily and stay at a job you don't even like, though you dream of going back to school and becoming a psychologist.

All of us desire some sense of security and safety, knowing that we have the ability to physically survive. We also want to feel loved, admired, and valued and that our life has relevancy, just like Jenna.

Anytime your desires or wants are threatened, or at least you believe they are threatened, your stress response is stimulated. If you find yourself faced with a challenge that reminds you of a hurtful memory, of a time when your wants or desires were endangered, your stress response will get triggered as well. The result can be an overactivated stress response that causes you to experience more physical, emotional, or psychological problems, like Jenna. In other words, your stress response is not just provoked by stressful situations, but also by underlying fears and beliefs that are based on past experiences.

When you address your triggers and the underlying negative beliefs that they are based on, you have a better chance of regulating the stress response, being able to maintain an enhanced peace of mind and healthier body. In essence, you are better able to assume power over your health and your life.

Being Aware That the Body Speaks

Feelings or sensations are the body's way of letting you know when it is out of balance and needs your help. When you are feeling tired, your body is letting you know you need rest; when you are hungry, that you need food; when you are cold, that you need to be warmer. In other words, feelings relate to your state of well-being, energy, stress level, mood, or disposition. If you can take a moment to pay attention, to listen to your body's whispers, you then might learn the language of your body, understand what your feelings mean and what your patterns are.

Your body has a unique way of speaking to you. Every one of your cells has the ability to communicate with others and ultimately with the neurons in your brain. Via neurotransmitters like serotonin and hormones like adrenalin or cortisol, cells report on the changes and challenges that are happening in your environment, both inside and outside of your body, inside and outside of each cell.

There are, for example, about a hundred million neurons lining your gut that enable you to "feel" the internal world of your gastrointestinal tract. According to Emeran Mayer, a professor of physiology, psychiatry, and biobehavioral sciences at the David Geffen School of Medicine at UCLA, these neurons are not just responsible for enabling you to digest food; they also direct your emotions.[1] Ninety-five percent of the body's serotonin lies in the gut.[2] Have you ever had that feeling of "butterflies" in your stomach when you were anxious? With anxiety, dropping serotonin levels change the activity in your gut and the electrical signals going from the gut to your brain, which cause you to feel "butterflies." This sensation is sending messages to the brain that you are in danger, so that the stress response will be activated. When your gut is healthy and feeling "happy," serotonin levels rise and signal your brain that all is well. That is how "comfort food" gets its name. Foods rich in fat and sugar temporarily stimulate serotonin levels to rise.

There are similar dense masses of neurons throughout your body. When messages are sent to the brain, it integrates the information from these areas with its database of memories and past experiences in order to make the executive decision that will ultimately move you into action. The action will be one that is meant to bring you relief and reward, so that you feel better.

Learning to Accept and Control
Your Need for Reward and Relief

When you feel better, it is because reward centers in the brain are stimulated and neurotransmitters like dopamine are released along with feel-good chemicals like endorphins and morphinelike substances. When you don't feel better, or rather if your bad feeling persists, neurotransmitter levels drop as the stress response keeps going into action. Rather than experiencing positive emotions, negative emotions prevail, so that your brain continues to motivate an action or behavior that will, at the very least, get you feeling better, even if it doesn't solve the problem. If you incur this same problem repeatedly, and you repeatedly use the same action or behavior to feel better or cope, it becomes a "bad" habit or a form of maladaptive coping. In other words, it is a behavior pattern that helps you cope, but that is not adaptive for health and for thriving.

For example, let's say that when you were a child your parents often fought. Perhaps you often experienced fear or anxiety. You did find that your parents seemed to be nicer to one another when you brought home good grades and ate everything on your plate. As an adult, you find that you cannot handle conflict very well, and when the going gets tough, you throw yourself into your work and you find solace in a pint of ice cream. Even though you realize you have become a workaholic with an ice-cream addiction, you do not know of any other way to feel as good, and you certainly don't have time to figure it out. Right now, the rewards you receive from work and ice cream are guaranteed.

Studies show that there exists a set of neural structures, including the ventral striatum, anterior insula, anterior cingulate cortex, and midbrain, that encode the subjective value of rewards.[3] This subjective value is different for everyone, as it develops over time and is also partially genetically wired. It is based upon how good you have felt or might feel when acquiring said reward.

In other words, your behavior is driven by your need for reward and relief and how bad versus how good you invariably might feel in the future. When the stress response is overactive, especially when your triggers have been activated and you are feeling really badly, you can safely bet your rational thoughts will get thrown out the window. The point here is that there really is no point in blaming or shaming yourself. What is called for here is both acceptance that you have a programmed tendency or pattern for dealing with fear or stress and knowledge that this programming can be rewired over time. It took years for the habits to form, after all. The good news is that it does not take years for reprogramming, though it does take a lot of practice. Until such time as the new tendencies kick in, you may fall into these habits again for a while. And that's okay.

Taking Responsibility for What You Can Change

Once you accept your behaviors and tendencies as wired, automatic responses that can be rewired, you can start taking responsibility for your role in either keeping them active or changing them. Being accountable involves understanding that your unhealthy habits are a result of fear and an underlying belief in inadequacy and that you have a choice of changing that belief. It involves understanding that this belief was formed long ago, that it is often a distorted perception of the situation and of yourself, and that, as long as you maintain it, the habits will persist.

For example, my patient Michael complained of having social anxiety. He abhorred going to social gatherings. At parties, he claimed he felt tongue-tied and awkward. When I asked Michael why he thought this happened to him, he explained that he felt he was stupid and had nothing interesting to say. When Michael said these words out loud, even he realized how outlandish they were. Michael was an avid reader. He skied competitively and participated in triathlons. He traveled the world on bird-watching trips, many of which he led. He was hardly "stupid and uninteresting." Michael admitted that this belief had its origins in his childhood, when the children in school teased him for being shy and quiet, a habit he developed after his father told him one too many times that he was stupid.

Many of us, like Michael, hold on to thoughts that are not based in truth; also known as cognitive distortions, these are neither logical nor accurate. Rather, the thoughts are founded on past negative experiences that were beyond our abilities to understand and make sense of. As a result, rather than developing the understanding that the situations were hurtful, hard, or "bad," we developed beliefs and assumptions that *we* were bad or in some shape or form "not enough."

Being aware of this distorted belief was the first step for Michael. The second step involved accepting that it was partially responsible for driving him to learn so much and excel at everything he put his mind to, but that it was no longer needed as a driving force for success. The third step involved understanding that his belief would only have power as long as he gave it power and that he had volition over how he continued to respond. Michael had to now acknowledge that he was in the driver's seat, and he had the choice to take the actions necessary to reprogram his beliefs, his physiology, and his behavior to get to healthy and happy.

The following is a list of a few common cognitive distortions, based on the work of Aaron Beck and discussed by David Burns in his book *Feeling Good: The New Mood Therapy,*[4] and examples of negative beliefs that may be behind them (examples, not absolutes):

- **All-or-Nothing Thinking:** You perceive the events in your life in absolute categories instead of as on a continuum. For example, if you believe that something is less than perfect, you see it as a total failure, validating your underlying belief that you are a failure in general. This can indicate that you have a fear of being inadequate, being a failure, or lacking value, so you focus on some kind of absolute solution to fix the problem. Michael, for instance, felt tongue-tied at parties and concluded that he was stupid rather than simply nervous in social settings.

- **Overgeneralization:** You view a negative event as a part of a continued pattern of negativity while ignoring evidence to the contrary, the fact that many things in your life are positive. You may use the words "never," "always," "all," "every," "none," "no one," "nobody," or "everyone" to support your belief that you don't and never will have or be enough. This can reflect a fear of failure or inadequacy; it can also stem from fear of loss (that if you are happy, it will be taken away). Michael equated his social anxiety with being stupid, overriding the evidence that he was clearly not stupid, as he managed to have a successful career and life.

- **Magnification or Minimization:** You make the negative bigger and the positive smaller; for example, you exaggerate the importance of a problem, making it much larger than it necessarily is. "Catastrophizing" occurs when you tell yourself you absolutely cannot handle a given situation, when the reality is that it is really just inconvenient. A tendency to make such problems so important can indicate your underlying fears of being inadequate, unimportant, or dispensable.

- "Should" Statements: You have a precise, fixed idea of how you or others should behave, and when these expectations are not met, you exaggerate how bad it is, which causes you to feel resentment, guilt, or unhappiness. You often use "should" or "must" statements. Such behavior can reflect your own feelings of inadequacy or fear that if anything is less than perfect, your sense of safety, security, or value is being threatened.

- Personalization: You hold yourself personally and entirely responsible for situations that are not totally under your control, or you blame others without acknowledging your role in the problem. Experiencing shame or blame can be pointing to feelings of low self-worth and the belief that somehow, consciously or subconsciously, you are a bad person. For example, you blame your children for your locking yourself out of the house, because they were fighting and upset you, though you were the one who forgot to take the keys.

The end result of these cognitive distortions and negative thinking is that you end up feeling badly, which is often followed by subsequent maladaptive behaviors and actions that usually make you feel worse.

Developing and Actualizing the Tools for Trust

The action steps involved in empowering your ability to be healthy and happy are varied and ultimately involve reprogramming your mind and body to perceive yourself differently in life—as a victor rather than a victim. From learning to rewire underlying beliefs, to developing positive expectancy, to improving lifestyle behaviors, to taking up meditation and healthy nutrition, the end result of your actions is developing an inner trust, in mind and body, that you have the power to heal and to overcome anything. When you develop the belief that you can react to stress in a constructive way and create your own toolbox for doing so—which involves listening to your body's whispers—you create greater resilience through trusting yourself and your ability to handle stress.

When you possess this inner trust, you are able to handle uncertainty and stress more efficiently, thus better regulating your stress response and the neurobiological mechanisms involved. You are more likely to be resilient and be able to:

- Face your fears.

- Keep your head clear so that you can problem-solve and fully appraise your situation.

- Keep up positive emotions and a positive outlook.

- Stay open to support.

- Feel competent in your actions.

- Maintain a sense of life's purpose and the ability to make meaning of your situation.

- Stay healthy and happy, with better emotional balance, improved sleep, and more calm and peace.

In addition, changing your perception and attitude from victim to victor will also be reflected in your body's physiology. When the stress response is less active, or down-regulated, the body may show:

- A decrease in heart rate and blood pressure.

- An improved metabolic rate.

- Less inflammation.

- Improved immunity.

- Lower levels of stress hormones like cortisol and adrenalin in circulation.

- More muscle relaxation.

- Improved mood.

- Enhanced memory.

- An improved ability to recuperate from the harmful effects of stress and to regain the natural ability to cope with additional stress.

Indeed, this latter factor should be underlined, as being able to successfully adapt to adversity, stress, or trauma is really the mark of resilience.[5] When you are resilient, adversity doesn't get you down physically, emotionally, or psychologically—at least not for too long, because you bounce back stronger and better and have an inner trust that you have the resources to handle anything.

There exists a myriad of action steps that can help you develop and cultivate this inner trust. Some of these actions you are well aware of, like regular exercise, healthy eating, and getting restful sleep. Other action steps may be new to you, as they stem from ancient or wisdom traditions, like developing a meditation practice or "opening your heart to experience love or oneness," a state that is opposite to the experience of fear and separateness. As you read through each chapter, you will learn concrete action steps and discover which ones work for you best.

The sciences of stress physiology, neuroplasticity, epigenetics, and positive psychology are actually playing catch-up with the time-tested theories and practices of ancient wisdom that have used the concepts of love and trust to heal the body for thousands of years. In fact, science shows us that oxytocin, the hormone involved in the formation of loving attachments and social bonding, is also implicated in our ability to trust. Research shows that oxytocin shapes the nerve circuitry of trust in the brain.

In a double-blind study conducted at the University of Zurich, researchers gave subjects intranasal oxytocin and studied their behavior and associated brain changes on fMRIs. Subjects in the oxytocin group showed no change in their trusting behavior after they learned that their trust had been breached several times, while for subjects receiving the placebo, trust decreased. This difference in trust adaptation was associated with a specific reduction in activation in the amygdala and other regions of the brain associated with the stress response.[6] "We now know . . . what exactly is going on in the brain when oxytocin increases trust," says lead researcher Thomas Baumgartner. "It seems to diminish our fears."[7]

What all the action steps have in common is that they offer outlets of relief for the stress response, enabling you to keep the response in better check, so that you can maintain a clear mind, positive expectancy, and a body that is full of vitality.

It is now *your* choice.

CHAPTER THREE

POWER Your Way to Health

Flow with whatever may happen and let your
mind be free. Stay centered by accepting
whatever you are doing. This is the ultimate.

—CHUANG TZU

believe I died climbing those stairs," John remembered as he contemplated the thought of climbing up the 199 steps at the Porter Square train station. "I need to climb those stairs again. I can't be scared of them anymore."

In November 2010 John found himself at the Porter Square train station in Cambridge, Massachusetts, on a day the escalator was not working. The alternative elevator had a long line, so he decided to walk up the 199 steep steps to the exit level.

The problem was that John had a "bad heart." He had a cardiomyopathy, a condition that caused his heart to be big, floppy, and essentially useless in pumping blood efficiently. His condition had progressed to the point that an internal cardiac defibrillator (ICD) had been implanted in his chest, which worked to shock his heart in case it stopped.

John climbed the 199 stairs only to find himself needing twenty minutes to catch his breath. By the time he arrived at the Chinese restaurant across the street, he collapsed before he had the chance to order. When he came to, he found himself lying on a gurney in an ambulance heading to Massachusetts General Hospital, alive only because his ICD had shocked his heart back to life.

While in the hospital bed, John was acutely aware that his heart would not be able to sustain too many more shocks. He needed a new heart, but he had to get in line, and the wait could be long. In the interim, he vowed to get stronger and someday conquer those stairs.

John was given a left ventricular assisting device (LVAD), a contraption that was attached to his heart on one end and on the other to a heavy external battery that he had to carry in a special case. The LVAD would now pump his heart, allowing him to live while he waited for a new heart. The wonders of modern medicine!

He also optimized his lifestyle habits and support system by changing his diet, walking a slow three miles a day, running a charity for the support of heart-transplant patients, and writing a blog and newsletter for his friends and supporters. He and I worked together on ways he could recognize the onset of his anxieties and worries. Together, we identified negative emotions and feelings that made him feel worse, which he sought to defuse as a way to help him quiet his mind and find balance within himself.

After several months, John decided to try again to conquer the Porter Square stairs. He was anxious. I instructed John that when his anxiety reared itself, he was to pause and focus on his breathing, while repeating the words "Sa, Ta, Na, Ma," Sanskrit chanting sounds that translate as "birth, life, death, rebirth." I explained that the meditation exercise would help quiet his mind, reduce his stress levels, improve his circulation, and allow the body to relax yet remain alert. It would also allow him to be better attuned to his body's signals, so he would know when to stop and when to keep moving.

After his next attempt at the Porter Square stairs, John said, to his surprise, "It was not bad. I stopped a couple of times, but I was going pretty fast. I was in the flow. I felt great!"

John isn't scared of those stairs anymore. Through this experience, he learned to strengthen his trust that he has the power to survive, thrive, and even get through the wait for a new heart. He discovered that he needed to pay attention to his body's signals, to rest when he was tired, spend time with friends to avoid feeling lonely, and honor the emotions he experienced as he wondered about the day when he wouldn't always feel so tired. His accomplishment—his learned ability to keep his mind quiet and his body in flow—continued to give him the strength to keep moving, despite his daily fears and frustrations.

Ten months later, he finally received a new heart. John knows now more than ever that he needs to continue practicing what he has learned, so that he has the *power* to give his new heart and himself a new life.

The POWER to Heal

Everybody has the power to heal. With the accumulation of stress, the body loses its ability to bounce back, as every system is taxed and overworked. In order to change the destiny of your health, you'll want to become more familiar with what "health" means to you and your body, so you can maintain your "bounce-back" abilities and gain power over your health and your life, as I described in the previous chapter.

From here on, therefore, you will learn how to use the word POWER as an acronym, as an actual guide that will enable you to truly heal and thrive. In this chapter I will explain to you the concepts that support the POWER acronym. Throughout the upcoming chapters, POWER will be used as an outline that will guide you to not only treat problems that may arise in the different systems of your body, but to prevent them from happening in the first place.

P.O.W.E.R.

PAUSE, so that you can clear and open your mind.

OPTIMIZE your awareness of the parts of the body and how they function.

WITNESS your own body's language and physiology, so that you can further your awareness and move into acceptance, understanding how your body speaks to you.

EXAMINE the deeper emotions and beliefs that are adding to your stress, furthering your awareness and acceptance, and moving you into accountability.

Develop action steps to **R**ELEASE negative habits and beliefs, **R**ELIEVE your body of stress, and **R**ESTORE power that will bring your mind and body into balance.

When you learn to become aware of and accept your body's signals and begin to listen to and understand what it is telling you it needs, you will make better choices, be more accountable for your actions and choices, and take action steps that enable you to take care of yourself in ways that truly help you to get healthy and happy.

The first step is to hit the pause button, to take a break from your busy life and ongoing thoughts. When your mind is busy and noisy, you can't hear your body's signals or be open to learning or processing new information.

PAUSE

Imagine you are engaged in one of your favorite activities—golf, tennis, dancing, singing, or skiing. Every movement is precise—the perfect swing, the perfect pirouette, the perfect C sharp, the perfect ski jump.

You are not thinking. Your mind and body are one unit. It feels like a dream. Smooth. No mistakes. In this moment, anything seems possible.

Then you begin to analyze and overthink every movement. You worry. Will you fail? Will you trip? Will your voice crack? Perhaps you remember that the last time you went skiing you fell, which causes you to fall. Like a toddler learning to walk, you act with hesitation rather than with confidence and ease. Your focus, timing, and coordination are way off the mark. Physically, emotionally, and mentally you expend more energy trying to perform than actually performing. Your mind has gotten in the way of your success.

This happens on an everyday basis. How much energy do you expend thinking, worrying, analyzing, and trying rather than simply being or doing? To the brain your fears and perceived obstacles represent unmanageable stressors. What does this mean? Normally, when the brain perceives a stress to be manageable, it will activate the stress response long enough to take care of the problem. If the stress is perceived to be unmanageable, the stress response will be activated incessantly. This means your heart continues to race, your blood pressure to climb, your digestive system to shut down, or the inflammatory response to heighten. On a daily basis, the persistent activation of the stress response can take a toll on the mind-body system, depleting your energy and ultimately the trust in your own abilities and strengths to manage uncertainty or handle a challenging task.

Wouldn't it be better to be like John climbing those stairs? He managed to overcome fears and other obstacles with more ease. When you empty your mind of its fears—fear that you might fail, that something bad might happen, that the outcome will not be what you expect—you can tap into your inner trust. When you quiet the mind, your inner trust can be heard. You become more centered and balanced within yourself, more relaxed and unattached, yet alert and engaged.

Try it for yourself.

POWER BREATHS

Breathe in deeply.

Then exhale, letting all the air out of your lungs, allowing all your thoughts to float out of your mind into the wind.

Breathe in.

Breathe out. Thoughts flow out of your mind into the earth.

Breathe in.

Breathe out. Thoughts flow out of your mind into the ethers.

Breathe in.

Breathe out. Empty the mind.

Breathe in. Breathe out.

Now listen, look, feel. Observe.

How did that feel?

The constant chatter in your mind is usually composed of thoughts that keep you stuck in memories of the past or worried anticipation of the future. The chatter can have you so caught up in yesterday or tomorrow that you miss the "now." If you are not in the now, you cannot really listen or be open for learning. You want to create a little void, a kind of openness, so that new perspectives, information, and possibilities can come in.

The key is to remember that, although disrupting thoughts always pop up, you don't have to pay attention to them or let them take over. Observe them and let them pass without too much emotion or judgment. This is a process of allowance, where you allow yourself to learn, to be open to the unknown, and to trust that there are always possibilities for growth, happiness, and health.

In his book *The Power of Now,* Eckhart Tolle describes many different ways to be present in the moment.[1] He outlines the importance of a quiet mind. Without a quiet mind, you miss out on the joy and happiness of the moment, devoting too much time and energy to thoughts of yesterday or tomorrow. When it comes to your health and well-being, your goal is to quiet your mind long enough to become fully aware of your body and its functions without fear or judgment—to simply be present in the moment, no matter what's going on.

In the PAUSE section in the following chapters, as you set the stage to learn with an open mind, you will learn about the anatomy of your body.

OPTIMIZE Your Awareness

When your mind is open, you widen your lens of perception and create a big picture for yourself of how your body works and why. Optimizing your awareness involves understanding how your body functions, what problems can arise, and why, so that you can prevent them from happening or getting worse. It entails not only getting a clear picture of the anatomy of your body, but also when medical attention is warranted. You will learn about the prevalence and incidence of problems in different areas of the body, risk factors, and causes as well as the "red flags"—the signs and symptoms that your body really needs medical attention sooner rather than later. This information is meant to guide you to take care of yourself, so that you can be at your optimal best.

WITNESS Your Physiology

Witnessing your physiology involves listening to and observing your body and how it speaks to you. You observe with an open mind without judgment. Nothing is good or bad; nothing is right or wrong. Witnessing has its roots in the Buddhist meditation practice called mindfulness, which is now a widespread secular practice. Mindfulness involves being in a moment-by-moment awareness of your thoughts, sensations, and feelings as well as of the surrounding environment. Thoughts tune into whatever you sense in the present moment, so that you can remain in the now.

The practice of mindfulness has many physical, psychological, and social benefits. Jon Kabat-Zinn created the Mindfulness-Based Stress Reduction (MBSR) program at the University of Massachusetts Medical School, a model now used to study and provide the many benefits of mindfulness in a variety of places, including schools, prisons, and hospitals.[2] Studies have shown that the practice of mindfulness meditation invigorates the immune system, improves positive emotions, reduces the effects of stress, and alleviates depression.[3] Other studies have shown that mindfulness can help tune out distraction and enable better focus and memory, which is exactly why this tool is used to "witness."[4]

By tuning out distractions and negative emotions, you can tune into the language, feelings, and memories of your mind and body. You also learn to reduce your stress-response reactivity, improve your mood, and cope more effectively with life's challenges.

EXAMINE Your Deeper
Emotions and Beliefs

When your mind is quiet, you can pay closer attention to the emotions and thoughts, beliefs, and memories that lie beneath physical sensations and feelings. When the body reacts with a physical sensation or discomfort, there are often emotional and psychological symptoms as well. Rather than trying to numb that discomfort with a medication, you can examine it more closely to uncover the underlying emotion.

Teachings from wisdom traditions can guide you to understand that different parts of the body are associated with a variety of emotions and beliefs. For example, the Vedic (Indian) chakra system and the five-element system from traditional Chinese medicine help us understand which belief or emotion may correspond with which symptom or part of the body. If, for example, you suffer from lung problems, the five-element system reveals that you may have experienced some loss or grief at some point, while the chakra system says heartache results from an imbalance within your heart chakra. Together, these systems teach that you may have some negative beliefs related to your sense of belonging and feeling loved and attached. As you read through each chapter, you will be given references to both systems. For now, this is what you want to know.

The five-element theory asserts that all things in nature and in the human body are made up of five elements that regulate cycles of growth and change—wood, fire, earth, metal, and water. The cycle of growth and change regulated by these elements is seen in all natural processes, including the seasons and human life. Each element has its own unique physical, emotional, and spiritual property, which is constantly moving and changing.

Each of the five elements is associated with particular organs that have both physiological and psychological functions. These are called organ networks. Each element is associated with a taste, a color, a sound, an emotion, and a season. All elements are present in all humans, though individuals are believed to have a tendency toward an imbalance in a particular element, which results in particular physical or emotional symptoms or behavior patterns. All the elements constantly interact with one another. Each element acts upon two other elements, nourishing one and controlling the other, similar to the relationship between a parent and a child.[5]

The knowledge of chakras dates back to 2000 BCE in India, where chakras were identified as centers or vortices of energy and consciousness that constantly spin or revolve, much like the sun. (In Sanskrit, *chakra* means "whirl" or "wheel.") Chakras are in constant movement, traversing space and time. In the body, there exist seven major chakras, interconnected by the spinal column and each emanating from a main nerve ganglion. Much as in the five-element system, each chakra is associated with certain organs and with physiological, physical, psychological, emotional, and spiritual functions. Each chakra correlates with specific colors, sounds, vibrations, and developmental stages of life.[6]

Ideally, each chakra is in balance, both with itself and with the other chakras. Chakras are like the individual circuits in the fuse box, which correspond to different areas of the house. The chakras essentially direct energy to different parts or aspects of your mind and body. When the chakras are in harmony, the circuits fire smoothly, and your mind and body function well.

Remember, these two systems are guides, not absolutes. Your body knows best what it needs, what you require for healing and strengthening. Through different examination exercises, you will learn how to do this for yourself.

RELEASE, RELIEVE, and RESTORE

Once you have taken a pause, opened your mind, optimized your awareness, identified the language of your body as well as underlying beliefs or emotions that warrant healing, you want to create outlets of release and relief, so that you can restore balance in your mind and body. You can imagine your body as a body of water behind a dam; you need outlets of relief to maintain the desired water level. These outlets make use of adaptive coping tools that you have at your fingertips should you choose to use them. They are adaptive in that they allow for regulation of the stress response and for reward and relief, which are beneficial to your health and well-being.

Throughout each chapter, you will be engaging in mindfulness practices that will help you shift out of the stress response into a more balanced state. You will also learn to identify your negative feelings, emotions, and beliefs as they contrast with your positive feelings, emotions, and beliefs.

You often don't know that you are feeling badly until you are feeling good. You also often don't appreciate feeling good until you have experienced feeling badly. This is what I refer to as learning by having contrasting experiences. When you have had the opportunity to experience both feeling good and feeling bad, which would you prefer to feel in the future? Now that you have experienced both, you have a choice.

For instance, you always have a choice about how you want to feel at any particular moment, even in a trying situation. You can choose to get upset and stressed about a challenging predicament, or you can choose to redirect your focus to positive thoughts, virtues, emotions, experiences, or imagery to transcend any negative thoughts and emotions. Perhaps you feel angry or worried, for example. You have the choice to focus on the object of your anger or worry, or you may choose to redirect your focus to something unrelated and more positive in an effort to shift your physiology and access positive thinking and emotions. You may try closing your eyes, taking a few slow, deep breaths, and focusing on the image of the smile of someone you love. Recall all the details of that smile—without judgment or repression. Just notice. As you breathe in and out, notice all the details and focus on the smile. If you concentrate on how the image makes you feel, you will become aware that you have shifted into a more positive state. You will also realize that you want to hold on to this wonderful feeling of joy and appreciation and that you are not experiencing negative thoughts and emotions simultaneously.

You have the option of making many choices. Do you want to feel rested or tired? Energized or sluggish? Strong or weak? Like you belong or are alone? Victorious or victimized? The list goes on, and there exists an even longer list of tools available to you to help you make the healthier choice, one that enables you to feel good and stay feeling that way. Each chapter focuses on lifestyle habits, with a particular emphasis on nutrition, exercise, and finding ways to build loving relationships that help you stay healthier and happier.

Sleep, for example, is essential for your physical, psychological, and emotional well-being. A lack of sleep takes a large toll on your health. One of the most important questions I ask my patients is, "How is your sleep?" When they answer, "Fine," I know I need to probe more deeply. So I ask, "Do you get a full eight hours sleep? Do you feel rested upon awakening? Are you tired during the day?" Invariably, the answers are "No, I am not rested upon awakening"; "Yes, I am tired during the day"; and, more often than not, "No, I am not sleeping eight hours a day." I point out that if it takes them more than an hour to fall asleep, that counts as insomnia, and yet if they fall asleep the second their head hits the pillow, that may mean they are sleep deprived. Even modest sleep deprivation of one or two hours affects your physiology, especially stress physiology.[7]

You've heard the saying, "You are what you eat." Nutrition plays a large role in regulating your stress response. Studies show that high levels of blood cortisol (as occurs with chronic stress) lowers homocysteine and vitamin B concentrations in the body.[8] Other studies reveal that the intake of vitamins, especially the B vitamins, positively effects mood and cortisol responses (which are abnormally elevated during stress).[9] Stress can deplete other mineral stores, including selenium, copper, and iron, which play a role in immunity, inflammation, and some aspects of metabolism.[10]

Are you aware of what you eat and how different foods make you feel? Drinking more than one cup of coffee a day robs your body of important minerals, notably iron. What's more, it can increase anxiety levels, activate your body's stress response, and keep you up at night.[11] If you learn to pay attention to your body and mind, you'll notice these things. For instance, you'll notice that eating too much sugar or white flour leaves you achy, tired, and irritable. Many of my patients, in fact, have noted that they experience negative symptoms like fatigue and indigestion immediately after eating such foods.

You are also meant to move, not sit for long periods. Every body has its own unique process. Some individuals require high-intensity cardiovascular exercise, while others respond best to gentle stretching exercise. Regardless, exercise is good for you. It is key in deactivating the stress response. Countless studies have shown the benefits of exercise. Exercise increases strength and flexibility; improves cardiovascular health, cognitive function, the levels of "good" cholesterol (high-density lipoprotein, or HDL), and bone density; decreases the risk for diabetes and for certain cancers like colon and breast cancer; and reduces symptoms of depression as effectively as antidepressants.[12] Exercise also releases tryptophan from albumin (a protein that acts as a transporter). Tryptophan is needed for the production of serotonin. The more serotonin you have in circulation, the better the effect on your mood and sleep.[13] A sedentary lifestyle, on the other hand, contributes to massive health problems, including diabetes, heart disease, and obesity. Along with knowledge from wisdom traditions, you will learn about movement and stretching, both of which strengthen different parts of your body.

As social beings, humans desire to be in groups. Social support is crucial to your health and well-being and can lower stress-response reactivity, largely because it releases hormones and peptides like oxytocin. Several studies have reported that social support facilitates coping and improves psychological and physical health.[14] Studies also confirm that strong, loving relationships improve physical health, while people who live in isolation or aren't part of a healthy social network are less healthy.[15]

For many, connecting does not just involve other individuals, but also being able to connect to something larger than themselves. Individuals with a strong spiritual belief system have been found to be healthier.[16] They often find more meaning in life and, as result, generally feel less helpless in adverse circumstances. Whether through organized religion or personal belief, these individuals have a more developed feeling of connectedness among themselves and to the world around them. Therefore they have more self-confidence, have a more positive outlook, and are better at problem solving.

I won't be advocating that you become more "religious." Instead, I will simply give you the tools that will enable you to connect to your own form of spirituality.

You can also experience a sense of deep connection by meditating or eliciting the relaxation response. Relaxation-response techniques stop the stress cycle at all levels. First described by Dr. Herbert Benson in 1971, the relaxation response is a state of deep rest brought about by focused attention on a simple mental stimulus in the form of a word, phrase, image, or prayer, such as "In peace, out tension," "Om," or "The Lord is my shepherd. . . ." Elicitation of the relaxation response is associated with reduced sympathetic nervous system activity, resulting in a lower heart rate, blood pressure, metabolic rate, respiratory rate, and muscle tension.[17] Dr. Benson coined the term after observing a hypometabolic state in people practicing Transcendental Meditation. With regular practice, the relaxation response decreases blood pressure in both untreated and treated patients with hypertension. It also decreases frequency of migraines in patients who regularly elicit the relaxation response.

Numerous studies have also confirmed that relaxation response reduces chronic pain, blood pressure, postoperative complications, insomnia and a person's dependency on sleep medication, levels of anxiety and depression in infertile women, premenstrual symptoms, and nausea and vomiting during chemotherapy.[18] Other studies have found that the relaxation response improves psychological well-being. Electroencephalogram (EEG) studies, for instance, show that people who practice the relaxation response exhibit a slow synchronization of alpha and theta brain waves. Alpha waves are related to a state of relaxed wakefulness and the ability to be creative and understand new concepts. When eliciting the relaxation response and alpha-wave synchronization occurs, your ability to be creative, think clearly, and take in new ideas improves.[19] In fact, emotional tension has been found to block the alpha rhythm and thus the ability to be creative and assimilate new concepts. Theta activity has been associated with emotional processes and the maturity of the mechanisms linking the cortex, thalamus, and hypothalamus. It has been correlated with a state of maximal awareness, deep insights, and intuition.

Even more exciting, recent studies have shown that regular elicitation of the relaxation response can even change genomic expression.[20]

Are you aware of what this implies? The way your DNA expresses itself can change for the better when you meditate regularly, which translates into better health and happiness for you.

Your goal now is to create a box of tools, an infrastructure, or outlets of relief that enable you to stay balanced and happy. No two individuals are alike, so pay attention to what techniques and recommendations work for *you*. Keep your mind open, learn, and see how you feel, and, remember, this toolbox will give you the POWER you need to change your health destiny.

CHAPTER FOUR

The Immune System

Your 24-Hour Security System

Your immune cells are like a circulating nervous
system. Your immune system in fact is a circulating
nervous system. It thinks. It's conscious.

—DEEPAK CHOPRA

A survey taken in Great Britain questioned more than two thousand adults about what they feared most. From a list that included Alzheimer's, debt, old age, getting stabbed, a plane crash, motor-neuron disease, a car accident, a heart attack, getting fired, losing their home, and cancer, the overwhelming majority chose cancer.[1]

There is cause to feel this way. After heart disease, cancer is the second most frequent cause of mortality in the United States.[2] Modern science is working to find a cure, but we still don't know how to fully prevent cancer or even anticipate when or whether it will happen. When DNA changes and mutates, a new cell is created with damaged DNA, which then gets copied and reproduced, usually faster than normal cells. As the mutated cells take over areas of the body, cancerous tumors form that attack those parts of the body. Some cancer cells are slow growing, but most quickly run rampant.

It seems to be almost impossible to determine ways to prevent DNA from mutating—but it's not. It's possible to prevent immune disorders or, at the very least, to create a strong immune system that can turn illness into an experience that passes rather than one that sticks around and maims.

Your immune system does more than just fight off the possibility of cancer. Your immune system is your twenty-four-hour security system that helps your body stay strong and healthy by preventing any sickness from taking over your body and your life. It defends against incoming toxins, bacteria, viruses, and other invaders. Indeed, the immune system's impressive armory includes antioxidants, proactive cells that seek out and neutralize dangerous free radicals.

A good way to understand what antioxidants are and why we need them is to think of the human aging process as similar to that of a car—over its life span, it will be driven over rough terrain and exposed to rain, possibly snow, and the strong rays of the sun. Without regular maintenance and tender loving care, the aging car can be prone to rust as a result of a process called oxidation. Oxidation also occurs with aging in the human body when it is exposed to different types of stress like cigarette smoke and processed foods. With oxidation, or "rusting," oxygen molecules that are missing an electron (free oxygen radicals) roam about your body looking for something to fill in the missing gap. As the free radicals have no real direction or aim, they end up crashing up against the cells of your body, causing general mayhem and, most of all, damage, like rust, if you will. Oxidative stress has been linked to a myriad of health problems, including cancer, heart disease, dementia, and autoimmune disorders.

Because antioxidants can prevent and treat this whole array of health problems, they may also extend your life.[3] In other words, your body has a natural ability to beat the aging process, heal damage, and prevent it from happening in the first place. Having said that, when the body is overtaxed and overstressed, the generation of free radicals can exceed the protective effects of antioxidants, resulting in oxidative stress and the damage associated with it.

When your immune system is tired and stressed, it cannot do its job well, and your body can start to manifest a whole host of problems— from heart disease and depression to autoimmune diseases and other inflammatory disorders. When it's strong, however, these problems are less apt to show themselves, and you are more likely to experience vibrancy and resilience. You have the ability to fight and win, even if you are exposed to sickness, and therefore positively influence your health destiny. This chapter will show you how to POWER up your immune system to help you fight disease and prevent it from happening in the first place. You will learn to:

- Press the PAUSE button and become acquainted with the anatomy and functions of the immune system.

- OPTIMIZE your awareness of what can go wrong with your immune system, the signs and symptoms to watch out for that tell you to get medical help, and what you can learn from wisdom traditions and their view of the immune system.

- Discover how your immune system may be subtly speaking to you as you WITNESS your physiology through guided exercises.

- EXAMINE the underlying emotions or beliefs that may be weakening the health of your immune system.

- Develop the tools that will help you RELEASE negative habits and beliefs that are taxing your immune system, RELIEVE your body of stress, and RESTORE power to your immune system.

PAUSE and OPTIMIZE Your Awareness of Your Immune System

Anatomy and Functions

Your immune system protects you every day—all day and all night—against bacteria, viruses, parasites, and toxins not just by fighting off these invaders, but by also keeping your body clean. It is composed of different kinds of cells, tissues, and organs as well as lymphatic vessels, which, like blood vessels, run throughout your entire body.

The cells of your immune system, or white blood cells, are called leukocytes. They are separated into two types: phagocytes, which eat up invaders, and lymphocytes, which help your body remember and attack invaders, should they return. Leukocytes are produced in your various lymphoid organs—the thymus, spleen, and bone marrow—and are housed in the lymph nodes and lymphoid tissues scattered throughout the body.

Your body is kept clean by a clear fluid, called lymph, that moves within tissues and through the lymphatic vessels. It is clear, as opposed to red, because it carries white blood cells instead of red blood cells. It travels through lymph nodes, where bacteria and viruses are filtered out by the lymphocytes that are housed there. If a lymph node swells, it usually means that there is active fighting and filtering happening. The lymph node that usually swells is the one that is draining the particular part of the body where an infection, foreign body, or group of bad cells is located, like the glands in your neck, which swell when you have a throat infection.

Your immune system is divided into two parts, the adaptive immune system and the innate immune system. You are born with your innate system, while the adaptive (sometimes referred to as "acquired") system develops over time, as you are exposed to diseases or immunized against them. [4]

Your innate immune system takes care of toxins or infectious agents that enter your blood or try to enter through your skin, mucous membranes, or stomach. The innate immune system is composed of physical barriers that are located throughout the body, including the skin and the respiratory, gastrointestinal, and genitourinary tracts. The immune cells in your respiratory tract, for instance, will mount an inflammatory response when you inhale cigarette smoke in an attempt to expel the smoke. This is why people violently cough the first time they smoke. The body knows it's harmful.

Your adaptive immune system, made up of T-cells and B-cells, a cascade of complements used to directly destroy foreign things, and antibodies, is designed to mount an even stronger attack than your innate immune system as well as keep a memory of past invaders. This part of your immune system has memory cells that keep track of invaders by remembering their specific signature, or the nonself pattern that is on the surface of these invader cells, or antigens, so that if you were to be exposed again, a very specific and deadly attack would ensue to completely eliminate the invasion before it gets going.

For example, let's say you have been exposed to the chicken pox. You experience flulike symptoms, develop a rash all over your body, and feel generally sick for a week or so, as your immune system mounts a general response to fight the virus (not specific to the virus). While this is happening, your adaptive immune system is "remembering" the signature of the chicken-pox cells, or antigens. If you are then exposed to the chicken pox virus again, your adaptive immune system will mount an attack with specific antibodies that are directed at the chicken-pox virus, so that it is eliminated immediately. This is why after being exposed once to the chicken-pox virus, you usually have protection against it for life.

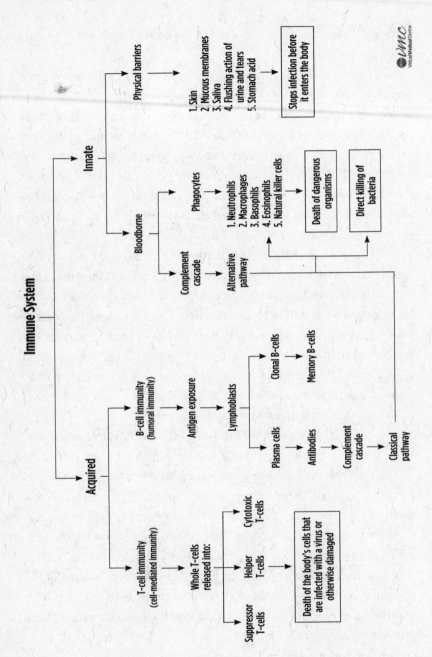

Immune System

Innate

Physical barriers

1. Skin
2. Mucous membranes
3. Saliva
4. Flushing action of urine and tears
5. Stomach acid

Stops infection before it enters the body

Bloodborne

Phagocytes

1. Neutrophils
2. Macrophages
3. Basophils
4. Eosinophils
5. Natural killer cells

Death of dangerous organisms

Complement cascade

Alternative pathway

Direct killing of bacteria

Acquired

B-cell immunity (humoral immunity)

Antigen exposure → Lymphoblasts

Clonal B-cells → Memory B-cells

Plasma cells → Antibodies → Complement cascade → Classical pathway

T-cell immunity (cell-mediated immunity)

Whole T-cells released into:

Suppressor T-cells

Helper T-cells

Cytotoxic T-cells

Death of the body's cells that are infected with a virus or otherwise damaged

Because the immune system is working around the clock, it can get taxed and lose its effectiveness. The good news is that your immune system can also be extremely resilient and can right itself too—that is, when you take care of it—even if it has been taxed.

Awareness of Immune Functions and Deficiencies

One of your immune system's primary functions is defense, and to perform this function adequately, it uses a powerful surveillance team that peruses the body for invaders like viruses, bacteria, free radicals, and toxins. Poor defense means more susceptibility to the ill effects of toxins, cancerous growths, or infection. Individuals with *immune deficiencies* have a difficult time getting over simple colds or recovering from even minor cuts and bruises. Examples of immune deficiencies include HIV/AIDS, hypogammaglobulinemia, and immunoglobulin A deficiency. In some cases, the body's defense system is overtaken by mutated DNA cells, resulting in different types of cancers.

On the flip side, your immune system could be overly defensive, so that it is hypersensitive and ready to mount an attack at the slightest provocation. With *allergic reactions,* the immune system's surveillance is on high alert and intolerant of substances that most other individuals are immune to or at least can tolerate. Examples include asthma and eczema. The surveillance system is also on high alert when it comes to *autoimmune disorders,* like rheumatoid arthritis (affects joints and sometimes organs), lupus (joints and organs), ulcerative colitis (the colon), Hashimoto's thyroiditis (the thyroid), and scleroderma (skin, joints, and organs). In these cases, the immune system sees your own tissue as an "invader" and specifically targets your own cells.

Why and How Deficiencies Happen

As I have discussed previously in this book, there is no single reason why disease happens. A lot of causes and risk factors are avoidable and correctable and, as is often the case, interconnected. Genetics play a role, but not all of the time. Nor is the role of genetics absolute. Although your genes and family history can play a role in increasing your risk of getting certain cancers, autoimmune diseases, allergies, and even immune deficiencies, this isn't always the case. Even though a disease may be caused by a genetic mutation, environmental factors often play a more significant role. In other words, your environment and what you put in your body greatly influence your immune functions.

Some immune deficiency disorders are purely genetic (primary), but others occur because the immune system has broken down as a consequence of environmental factors. These environmental factors include medications like steroids or chemotherapy, infections like HIV, or overexposure to radiation from ultraviolet rays of the sun.

Indeed, a connection has been found between exposure to a virus and the increased risk of developing autoimmune disorders, deficiencies, or allergies. Being exposed to viruses or bacteria may also increase the risk for cancer. This is often the case with individuals exposed to human papillomavirus. They are at an increased risk of getting cervical cancer. Similarly, individuals exposed to helicobacter pylori bacteria are more susceptible to stomach cancer.[5]

Your environment, what you do with your body, and what you put in it greatly influence how your immune system functions. Smoking and a diet high in fat and processed food can increase your risk for things such as lung or stomach cancer, heart disease, diabetes, depression, and other immune disorders, including autoimmune disorders.[6] The 2012 annual report on the occurrence of and trends in cancer in the United States, for instance, highlighted the increased cancer risk with obesity and lack of sufficient physical activity (less than 150 minutes of physical activity per week).[7] According to the National Cancer Institute at the National Institutes of Health, obesity alone is associated with increased risk of cancers of the esophagus, breast, endometrium, colon, rectum, kidney, pancreas, gallbladder, and likely more.[8] Ultraviolet light exposure to the skin can increase the risk of skin cancer, while alcohol can increase the risk of cancer in the throat, liver, esophagus, colon, breast, and rectum.[9]

A variety of immune disorders are connected to a diet devoid of necessary vitamins and minerals, which creates deficiencies in the body, including a deficiency in vitamin D.[10] Essential vitamins and minerals are called "essential" because they are vital for your body's functions, including, but not limited to, metabolism, digestion, muscle function, mental acuity, immune strength, and cardiovascular performance. Deficiencies, therefore, can have marked negative consequences on your immune system. Vitamin D, for instance, has a direct and indirect ability to regulate the immune system, stimulating immune cells to multiply or differentiate (change from a general into a more specific form). Lack of vitamin D has been implicated not only in conditions involving the bones, but also in autoimmune disorders and deficiencies.[11]

Current studies also suggest that overuse of antibacterial soaps, or too much hygiene, if you will, is wiping out much of the natural bacteria we need for healthy immune functioning, so that individuals are now more prone to allergies and autoimmune disorders.[12] Although some bacteria are harmful to your body, many are necessary for protecting you against toxins and for helping your immune system in its functions. For instance, you have bacteria in your gut lining producing organic acids that kill other bacteria that can cause harm to the intestines.

Your take-home message here is that there is plenty you can do to POWER up your immune system, especially when it comes to diet, exercise, and how you choose to take care of yourself. If you do not take heed, though, disease can—and will—take over.

The Gruesome Facts

Since the problems that can arise due to malfunctioning of the immune system are so vast and broad, it is difficult to talk about the causes and risks for all possible problems. Some important facts:

- An immune deficiency affects upward of 1 million Americans and 10 million people worldwide, according to statistics compiled by the American Academy of Allergy, Asthma, and Immunology.[13]

- An estimated 50 million Americans, approximately one in five, suffer from some type of allergy. The prevalence has increased among all age, race, and gender groups since the 1980s.[14]

- Allergies are the fifth leading cause of chronic disease in the United States in all age groups.[15]

- The National Institutes of Health estimate up to 23.5 million Americans—and counting—suffer from autoimmune disease.[16]

- Autoimmune disease is one of the top ten leading causes of death in girls and women up to sixty-four years of age.[17]

- About 1,660,290 new cancer cases are expected to be diagnosed in 2013.[18]

- Cancer remains the second most common cause of death in the United States, accounting for nearly one out of every four deaths.[19]

Red Flags That Tell You to Seek Help

The most life-threatening allergy-related problem that can occur is anaphylaxis, a rapid and extreme allergic reaction. Anaphylaxis involves a variety of symptoms, including hives, flushing, sweating, swelling (particularly around the eyes and mouth), a runny nose, itchy or red eyes, shallow breathing, an accelerated heart rate, a sudden drop in blood pressure, stomach cramps, vomiting or diarrhea, and in some cases seizures.

These are life-threatening symptoms! Call 911 immediately, even if the symptoms go away at first. Some individuals experience a second phase eight to seventy-two hours after the initial attack. If you have had this experience before, make sure you check with your doctor to uncover what is causing the allergy and always carry an epinephrine auto-injector (an EpiPen), which will immediately help stop the constriction in your airways and bring up your blood pressure.[20]

Other symptoms and signs that you want to be wary of, as they often point to cancer or other types of immune deficiencies, are:

- Unexplained weight loss, perhaps 10 pounds over a month without a change in diet or exercise

- Continued and unexplained abdominal or pelvic pain

- Abnormal bleeding, in between menses for women, or from any other part of the body

- A marked change in bowel movements, blood in the stool, indigestion, or abdominal pain

- Skin changes, such as a mole or red, chafed skin around the breast

- Persistent difficulty swallowing

- Persistent coughing, over three to four weeks

- Persistent pain in one or more parts of the body

- Enlarged or swollen glands bigger than 0.4 inches or ones that do not get smaller after several weeks

- Enlarged or swollen glands that are persistent and not associated with other symptoms or signs of infection such as a runny nose, fever, or sore throat

- New growths like a changing mole or a lump in the breast, especially ones that feel hard to the touch (versus soft), seem fixed in one place (can't be grabbed completely with the fingers), or feel as though they have irregular borders

- Unexplained fatigue, night sweats, or persistent fevers

- White patchy growths in the mouth

What Wisdom Traditions Have to Say

Not all wisdom traditions address the immune system specifically. They do, however, address the body's defense mechanisms, the need for the body and these mechanisms to be strong to fight off invasion by disease-causing agents, and how necessary they are in maintaining adaptability and homeostasis. In traditional Chinese medicine, for instance, *nei wei qi* is translated as "internal defensive life force" and *zheng qi* as the "antipathogenic factor"; when strong, these prevent invasion or deficiencies from happening. *Vyaadhiksamatva,* a term in Ayurveda, means "resistance" (*ksamatva*) against "disease" (*vyaadhi*). In this tradition, the goal is to maintain strong resistance, the integrity of the body's tissues, and an individual's bioenergy (called *dosha*). The stronger the body's tissues and the life force or energy (*oja*) within these tissues, the stronger the resistance to disease.

Whether it is traditional Chinese medicine, Ayurveda, or another wisdom tradition, the concept of immunity is intertwined with improving the body's energy; reinforcing an individual's life force and constitution; strengthening the integrity of the mind, body, and spirit; and enabling harmony and balance to exist within the individual and between the individual and the environment. This is accomplished through nutrition, exercise, following the cycles of nature, avoiding harmful foods or activities, and maintaining positive spiritual beliefs and practices that help an individual better develop balance and physical, psychological, and spiritual integrity. A resilient immune system thus is found in an individual who has a robust constitution and a healthy genetic makeup, who lives in accordance with nature, taking in wholesome foods and moving regularly, who has a strong mind focused on positive thinking, and who has a meditation practice through which to be able to disengage from disturbing thoughts and senses and instead connect with self-awareness and inner knowing.

If you pay attention to the studies connecting poor nutrition, lack of exercise, and environmental toxins with disorders of the immune system, you will note that wisdom traditions and modern medicine are fairly aligned when it comes to powering up the immune system. These are the takeaway themes:

- Develop a robust constitution.

- Develop strong integrity, in mind, body, and spirit.

- Foster durable defense and resistance systems to ward off harm.

- Maintain balance and harmony within the body and with others and nature.

As you move forward and learn to POWER up your immune system, think about your own lifestyle behaviors and choices as well as your beliefs and attitudes and ways they could possibly compromise your immune system. Think about the ways you might be putting unnecessary stress on your immune system. Are you getting adequate sleep? Are you providing your body with the nutrients it needs? Do you feel weak when it comes to saying no to people or food, or yes to your own needs?

WITNESS the Physiology of Your Immune System

The process of witnessing involves quieting the mind, so that you can pay attention to even the subtlest signs of fatigue, allergy, or weakness. This also allows you to notice the contrast between when your life force is vibrant and robust and when it is not. You can become aware of the contrast between your desire to stay awake and your body's desire to sleep or between your mind's desire to eat a donut and your stomach's call for liquids. This exercise is meant to awaken you to notice imbalances that warrant correcting, so that you can become healthier and stronger.

AWARENESS EXERCISE

Breathe in, breathe out. Bring your awareness to your mind. How tired is your mind? Observe.

Breathe in, breathe out. Focus on your throat. How much stress or strain is in your throat? Observe.

Breathe in, breathe out. Bring your awareness to your heart. Do you feel a sense of heaviness or strain in your heart? Perhaps a sense of fatigue? Observe.

Breathe in, breathe out. Focus on your solar plexus / stomach. Stress, strain, heaviness there? Observe.

Breathe in, breathe out. Focus on your sacral or pelvic area. Stress, strain, heaviness there? Observe.

Breathe in, breathe out. Focus on the base of your spine. What do you feel? Observe.

Breathe in, breathe out. Focus on your arms and legs. How tired are they? Observe.

Now ask yourself these questions:

Do the foods I eat make me feel strong or tired?

Does the amount or quality of sleep I get help me feel nourished?

How much stress can I tolerate or withstand? Can I handle loud noises or rude behavior? Do I stay calm, or do I tend to overreact easily?

Do the people in my life help me feel supported, so that I can handle challenges?

Do I have enough strength in me to get through the challenges in my life?

Do I feel safe and provided for?

Do I feel loved for being who I am?

Do I often feel I have to defend myself or my point of view?

Do I feel weighed down by life's responsibilities?

When you ask these questions, notice what you feel and where you feel it. For example, you may feel that you are not truly loved for being who you are or that you are not supported by others, and there's a feeling of strain or constriction in your stomach or solar plexus or in your chest. Perhaps you really don't feel safe, and you experience tension in your lower back, or you feel overburdened by responsibility, and feel tension or fatigue in your neck and shoulders.

EXAMINE Your Deeper Emotions and Beliefs

Your ability to trust that you have internal and external resources to manage life and its curveballs is tantamount to ensuring that the balance, health, and well-being of your mind and body stay intact. If for any reason you do not trust that your needs will be met or that you have the necessary resources to handle adversity, your stress response will be overactivated, meaning your immune system will be too, until such time, that is, that it burns out or loses its ability to stay balanced. Unmet needs—such as your need for food and shelter, your need to feel you belong, to feel you are relevant, worthy, or loved—can lead to an immune system that is tired and burned out from fighting all the time. Intuitively trusting that your needs can be taken care of now and in the future can reduce stress-response reactivity and lessen some of the allostatic load, both of which will enable you to be more in the flow of your life, like a Zen master.

Perhaps you can look deeper into your body's signals to see what requires your attention. The area of fatigue or tension you noted in the previous exercise is showing you where you may be weak. Maybe there is a message for you there.

When examining and asking yourself the questions below, notice the intensity of the emotion that comes up. Rate the intensity on a scale from 0 to 10, where 0 means you feel nothing and the thought/answer is untrue, and 10 means you feel an extreme amount of fear or anger and the thought/answer rings very true. You may wish to write down your answers.

GOING DEEPER EXERCISE

Identify the question or questions from the witnessing exercise to which you had the most intense reaction.

Close your eyes, breathe deeply, and bring your awareness back to the area of your body where you experienced the response. Ask yourself what situation comes to mind that supports this feeling? For instance, ask your body to show you an example when you were not supported or valued or you had to defend yourself.

You may ask yourself one of the following questions as you observe the story or image that comes forward.

Defense:

Why is this situation causing me to feel I have to defend myself? Do I feel attacked?

How long have I been defending myself? When did it start?

Am I feeling supported or do I feel alone?

Surveillance:

Am I always on guard? Why?

Can I trust people? If not, why not? What am I scared of?

Integrity and Harmony:

Do I often feel that my integrity is in question?

What do I do when I feel as though my balance is being threatened? What or who threatened my balance or sense of harmony and why?

You may notice as you pay attention to your emotions and the answers to the questions that your beliefs around feeling supported and your ability to trust that your needs will be met come forward. You may notice you often feel shame or that your past has taught you never to trust anyone. Look closely at who you are really attacking when you are angry or hurt. Are you attacking yourself? Are you blaming others for your misfortune?

Take your time to write out your answers, thoughts, and experiences and see what sort of pattern emerges.

RELEASE, RELIEVE, and RESTORE

Have you discovered anything new? Are you ready to build a robust constitution, strengthen the integrity of your immune system, and restore harmony and balance?

Releasing and Restoring

Now that you have uncovered emotions, beliefs, or stories that can be weakening your body, you can work on releasing them. The following exercise involves "emptying" the mind and body of this negativity and filling yourself up with the "breath of life" and all that is nurturing and positive. This exercise shares some similarities with many *qi gong* (literally "energy work" or, rather, "working with the life energy") exercises from traditional Chinese medicine, which help you strengthen your life force and vitality. You can practice this relaxation exercise on a daily basis to lower your stress-response activity and improve your mood, your immune system, and your ability to cope.

BUILDING YOUR LIFE FORCE MEDITATION

Close your eyes, and begin your breathing, counting to three as you breathe in and to five as you breathe out.

Bring your awareness to your mind. As you exhale, allow all the thoughts in your mind to be released into the earth, wind, or ethers.

Empty the mind for five or more breath cycles.

Then move your awareness to the parts of the body, relaxing and emptying each of tension in this order: throat, chest, solar plexus (above your belly button), lower abdomen/pelvic area, and entire spine, letting all tension and negativity drain out of the base of your spine. Do five or more breath cycles for each area.

Then, as you inhale, imagine you are breathing in the breath of life, the life force of the universe, so that it gathers in the base of your spine after five cycles of breath.

Then, as you inhale, allow the life force to move up your spine to the top of your head.

As you exhale, the life force will move through your mind and the center of your being and then come back to the base of your spine.

Circulate the life force at least three times, then notice how you feel.

Moving Your Body

If you are living a predominantly sedentary lifestyle, it can translate to a sluggish and sedentary immune system. Studies show that regular moderate exercise increases your leukocyte levels. This just means a fast walk for thirty minutes a day, and it does not have to be all at once. It can be cumulative. We now know that exercise increases strength and flexibility, improves cardiovascular health and cognitive function, decreases the risk for certain cancers like colon and breast cancer and reduces symptoms of depression as effectively as antidepressants.[21] Not only does physical activity help lower stress-response reactivity; it can also boost your immune system, even as you age.[22]

There is no "right" form of exercise. In fact, if you exercise at all, you're already headed in the right direction. For individuals who "burn out" or demonstrate signs of a suppressed immune system, I do not recommend strenuous exercise initially, as this will make you feel worse and further suppress your immune system. Instead, I recommend gentle exercises, such as walking, water aerobics, stretching, yoga, or tai chi. Otherwise, do what you enjoy.

Tips for Getting More Nature Time

- Spend twenty to thirty minutes a day, if possible, being active in nature.

- Put a plant in the room you spend the most time in.

- Exercise outdoors.

- Consider gardening.

- Spend time getting good sunlight for the vitamin D (about fifteen minutes a day), unless contraindicated by your doctor.

Here are some tips for exercise to POWER the immune system. These exercises also serve as the basis for strengthening all systems of the body:

- Walk for twenty to thirty minutes a *day* at a moderate pace (you can carry on a conversation).

- Aim for seventy-five minutes per *week* of high-intensity exercise (you cannot carry on a conversation).

- Play sports in a relaxed manner. Have fun!

- Do gentle exercises such as tai chi or yoga.

- Don't drive; walk whenever you can.

- Pay attention to how you feel before, during, and after exercising.

Healing and Reviving in Nature

If you are going to exercise, try to exercise outdoors. New research points to the benefits of nature in boosting your immune system. Ancient healers, including Greek physicians, used aromatic plant chemicals to stimulate or to sedate. Today, we find this ancient healing modality in aromatherapy, where plant aromas are used to enhance relaxation or offer other healing benefits. New science is confirming the benefits of aromatherapy—rosemary and lemon oil, for instance can influence the brain by stimulating it, while lavender and rose oil can calm.[23]

How does aromatherapy work? Scientists have long recognized the nasal passage as a potential area for administering medication, because it is a direct route to the brain. We have this passageway for a reason; most likely it was so that nature's aromas could have their various ef-

Plants Used in Aromatherapy and Their Benefits

Lavender: a mild sedative with a calming effect; associated with improved mood, cognitive performance, and stress reduction

Rosemary: associated with improved mood, performance, and stress reduction

Peppermint: associated with increased alertness and memory

Lemon balm: associated with antidepressant effects and stress reduction

Jasmine: an anti-spasmodic, sedative, and aphrodisiac; associated with antidepressant effects

fects on our brain. Nature provides a multitude of chemicals that provoke our olfactory (nasal) senses; many of them can balance mental outlook and energy.

Your sense of smell may or may not detect these chemicals, but they still have their effect. Some chemicals stimulate brain activity, while others relax or sedate the brain. Some plants give off volatile organic compounds, called phytoncides, that serve to protect them from invading bacteria and other aggressors; they have an effect on humans as well. Some experimental studies have shown that phytoncides produced by trees can lower the production of the stress hormone cortisol, lower anxiety, and reduce blood pressure.[24] The higher the level of phytoncides in the air, the more anticancer cells can be produced. According to numerous studies in Japan, a weekend *shinrin-yoku* trip (walking a mile and a half twice a day in a forest) raised natural killer-cell activity (fighting by immune cells) by 40 percent; a month later levels were still 15 percent higher than before the walking trip.[25]

Studies also show that you are more likely to exercise if it takes place outdoors.[26] It has been found that "green" improves your mental state whether you realize it or not. You may notice, however, that when you do exercise outdoors, you are less likely to cramp and experience fatigue or negative thoughts. In fact, researchers at Texas State University have found that athletes' performances improved when surrounded by more green space.[27]

Resting and Restoring by Getting Some Z's

During sleep is the best time for your brain—and the rest of your nervous system—to rest. While you sleep, your cortisol levels drop and your body naturally releases hormones, most notably the all-important growth hormone.[28] Growth hormone is a protein hormone that plays a major role in growth and in protein, fat, and carbohydrate metabolism. Deficiencies in growth hormone may present with such symptoms as fatigue, loss of muscle mass, weight gain, and feelings of anxiety, depression, or sadness. Getting more sleep may alleviate these symptoms. In addition, sleep activates the body's T-cells, which accelerates the natural healing process.

Impaired sleep affects memory and the ability to process information and remain fully alert. So imagine how this translates to the effectiveness of your immune system. As I mentioned in the previous chapter, even moderate sleep deprivation can lead to inflammation as both the stress response and your immune system are activated.[29]

Fortunately, a variety of methods can improve sleep:

- Practice progressive muscle relaxation. Tense each muscle group for five seconds and then allow those muscles to relax for thirty seconds. Start from the soles of your feet and work your way up to the top of your head.

- Elicit the relaxation response, especially before sleep.

- Exert stimulus control. Go to bed only when you are sleepy, awakening at the same time every morning, and avoid napping. Use your bed only for sleep or sex. Keep the bedroom atmosphere quiet, dark, and at a comfortable temperature, and avoid fluids after 8 P.M.

- If you are restless, get out of bed and do some other kind of activity until you're sleepy.

- Avoid food and drinks containing caffeine, sugar, or alcohol before bed.

- Add vitamins or supplements like melatonin or magnesium, if approved by your physician, or use aromatherapy to promote sleep.

- Exercise regularly during the earlier hours of the day.

You may also need to let your pet sleep in another room or on the floor, and your partner who snores may need to move to a different room. The good news is that you can "catch up" on your sleep loss by taking naps. However, for those individuals who have a hard time falling asleep, naps are not recommended. In general, naps should be limited to about twenty-five minutes.

Getting Power from Nutrition

As you have learned, carrying those extra pounds puts your immune system at risk. Eating foods that provoke the immune response to increase inflammation in the body also taxes the system. You evolved living in nature, so your body is designed to break down foods that are natural and familiar to your system. Taking in refined sugars, refined grains, processed foods, artificial sweeteners (and therefore added chemicals), trans fats and vegetable oils, meats from animals fed refined grains, and an excess of alcohol—all can provoke a heightened inflammatory response, make your immune system work harder because it has to put more effort into breaking down something foreign and unnatural, and wipe out bacteria living in the gut that normally promote metabolism and reduce inflammation.

In general, you want to follow a diet rich in monounsaturated and polyunsaturated fats (versus trans fats), lean protein, vitamins, minerals, enzymes, antioxidants, and, yes, bacteria or microorganisms that your body needs to thrive, all of which boost the power of your immune system.

ANTIOXIDANTS: Pump up the immune system with foods rich in antioxidants! Many delicious foods are loaded with natural antioxidants, which neutralize or rid the body of dangerous free radicals. Brussels sprouts, broccoli, tomatoes, grapefruit, cauliflower, cabbage, dark leafy greens, lemons, and limes have antioxidant properties and help reduce the risk of certain cancers. Blueberries are loaded with antioxidants called anthocyanins, as are red grapes. You can spice up your meals and add antioxidant value with herbs and spices like oregano, black pepper, turmeric, cinnamon, and cloves.

I personally like to get a good dose of chicoric acid on a daily basis, another natural antioxidant found in dark green lettuce, basil, chicory root, and dandelion greens. New research shows that chicoric acid can help with depression, as it appears that chicoric acid can raise the levels of "feel good" molecules or neurotransmitters (like dopamine and serotonin) and lower levels of stress hormones like cortisol.[30] I recommend throwing basil, dandelion greens, deep green lettuce, and chicory root into one big salad along with fresh blueberries. It is quite the antioxidant treat!

ESSENTIAL VITAMINS AND MINERALS: It is safe to say that pretty much all vitamins are needed to support your immune system. The ones to focus on include vitamins C, A, K, E, B5, B6, B12, B1 (thiamin), B2 (riboflavin), and folic acid.

Vitamin C is an immune stimulant and also functions as an antioxidant, as it supports healing and promotes healthy T-cell functioning. Good sources of vitamin C include citrus fruits and dark leafy greens like kale, broccoli, collard greens, Swiss chard, mustard greens, and asparagus.

The B vitamins are also essential for a powerful immune system, as B5 helps promote antibody production, B6 and folic acid promote T-cell functioning, B1 and B2 support the antibody response, and B12 supports T-cell and phagocyte functions. Good sources of the B vitamins, including folic acid, are whole grains, dark leafy greens (especially turnip greens and spinach for folic acid and B6) and other vegetables like cauliflower. Sources of B12 include salmon, tuna, sardines, cod, lamb, beef, scallops, and shrimp.

Vitamins A, E, D, and K all share the same property of being fat-soluble vitamins. While vitamin E functions as an antioxidant and as support for the inflammatory response, vitamin A supports both antibody and T-cell function. As you have learned, vitamin D is known to support immune system health, and deficiencies have been associated with an increase in autoimmune disorders and some cancers. Vitamin K is necessary for the clotting cascade to work properly, which is especially important in response to injury and in the healing process after injury. Vitamins A and E can be found in dark leafy greens like Swiss chard, mustard greens, and turnip greens. Vitamin A is also abundant in carrots, sweet potatoes, and asparagus. Sources of vitamin D include eggs, shrimp, and cod. Sources of vitamin K include cauliflower, spinach, and asparagus.

Have you noticed the common theme of dark leafy greens? Greens such as kale, collard greens, and spinach not only contain important vitamins and minerals, but also have antioxidant properties.[31]

You can't go wrong with eating green vegetables. You can also add in fruits and vegetables that have a deep color, like red, orange, or purple, because they are high in antioxidants, vitamins, and minerals like zinc, iron, copper, selenium, manganese, and magnesium. Zinc supports and stimulates the immune system. Both iron and copper support the immune system to fight infection. Magnesium, a mineral notoriously low in the general population (because it is a surrogate marker of eating green foods), is needed for the production and function of immune cells, and low magnesium is connected to a host of ailments, including allergic reactions and susceptibility to viral and bacterial infections.[32]

Dark leafy greens like spinach, kale, and mustard greens are good sources of iron and copper as well as zinc. Zinc and copper can also be found in some mushrooms, cashews, quinoa, and lentils. Sources of manganese include spinach, brown rice, pumpkin seeds, soybeans, pineapple, and oats, while selenium can be found in shellfish, tuna, sardines, salmon, cod, turkey, lamb, beef, and tofu.

FAT AND PROTEIN: Salmon, mackerel, lake trout, sardines, bluefish, albacore tuna, and fresh herring are not just great sources of some vitamins and minerals; they are also rich in omega-3 oil, an essential fatty acid that helps the body create the prostaglandin PGE2, an anti-inflammatory chemical that may decrease the risk of certain cancers.[33] Other sources of omega-3 fatty acids include flaxseed, walnuts, and almonds. Conjugated linoleic acid (CLA) is a fatty acid with strong anti-oxidant properties that is found in grass-fed animal meat.[34]

Grass-fed animal meat, walnuts, fish, and many of the other food sources mentioned also boost the immune system because of their protein content. Protein is essential for the growth and repair of your body's cells. A deficiency can lead to depletion of immune function and a slowing down of antibody production. Some preliminary studies show that supplementing with the amino acids arginine and glutamine can improve wound healing, including diabetic foot ulcers, as they stimulate the immune system.[35] Protein sources that support your immune system can therefore include eggs, fish, shellfish, grass-fed animal meats, legumes (like lentils, hemp seed, and soybeans), and grains such as quinoa, and amaranth. Good sources of protein, minerals, and vitamins like A and B6 for vegetarians include quinoa, which contains such amino acids as lysine and isoleucine, and amaranth, which provides a complete set of amino acids.

GUT CARE: Taking care of your gut supports your immune system. Sixty percent of your immune system exists in the lining of your gastrointestinal tract. These immune cells work hard to prevent invading organisms or damaging molecules from getting into your body. For this reason, it is important to maintain the gut barrier intact. Omega-3 fatty acids support the membranes of gastrointestinal cells, while vitamin A supports the production of mucus, which lubricates and cleanses. Your gut especially benefits from hosting bacteria that live naturally in the intestinal environment. These microorganisms aid in digestion and absorption of nutrients and keep the immune system in balance. Introducing foods into your meals that are high in these bacteria has been found to boost the natural bacteria in the gastrointestinal tract and reduce inflammation.[36] Such foods include kefir, miso, kimchee, olives, pickles, sauerkraut, or yogurt that is very low in sugar.

NUTRITION TIPS:

- Avoid inflammatory foods, which include simple or refined sugars or carbohydrates, too much caffeine and alcohol, trans fats, and processed foods.

- Eat more greens, legumes, and other vegetables.

- Eat foods rich in omega-3 essential fatty acids.

- Eat high-quality protein sources.

- Eat berries, spices, and herbs that are plentiful sources of antioxidants, vitamins, and minerals.

- Add fermented foods to your nutrition plan.

- Add a supplement if you cannot get a food source in your diet or if you note a deficiency. Check with your health-care provider to ensure that there are no contraindications for you.

Harmony Through Social Support and Love

Having strong relationships and a good social network is important to your immune system. Several studies support the idea that people who feel connected to friends—whether it's a few close friends or a large group—have stronger immunity than those who feel alone.[37] In one study, college freshmen who were lonely had a weaker immune response to a flu vaccine than those who felt connected to others.[38] Another recent study found that isolation changed the immune system on a cellular level: being lonely affected the way some genes that controlled the immune system were expressed.[39]

A strong social network helps you feel good about yourself and your life and stronger in the face of adversity. Knowing someone has your back means you feel more secure and empowered, which invariably means the cells of your body do too. This is a key component in changing your health destiny.

Some ways to build support for a healthy immune system include:

- Regularly meet with friends or family to socialize, talk, or connect.

- Participate in a church, temple, or preferred spiritual organization, if this interests you.

- Allow yourself to receive help from others, including your friends, family, counselors, and health-care providers.

- Join an interest group, like a book club, an outing club, or a "play group." A wonderful source is www.meetup.com, which offers a wide variety of interest groups in your area. You are bound to find something that suits you where you can meet like-minded or interested people.

- If you like pets, get one or borrow one!

- When you need a hug, simply ask.

CHAPTER FIVE

Opening Your Heart and Reclaiming Your Health

Hearts will never be made practical until they are made unbreakable.

—THE TIN MAN, *THE WIZARD OF OZ*

Why are you crying, Maia?"

"Because my heart hurts."

"Why does your heart hurt?"

"Because I miss my mommy."

"She's just out for the night. She will be here when you wake up in the morning."

"Oh."

"Does your heart still hurt?"

"Nope," she grinned. "Good night, Auntie. I love you."

It may not be this easy to mend a "hurt" heart when you are an adult or have a medical condition, but it is possible.

I can still recall the pain I felt in my heart after the end of one of my most significant relationships. One minute my heart was open, I felt as if I were flying high, bristling with love and joy, and the next minute, I could only feel pain; I wanted to crawl into a fetal position and withdraw from the world. My heart went from feeling full and whole to broken and incomplete. I felt tired and withdrawn, unable to think clearly or focus. Yet I also longed to love once more, and to allow that crack in my heart to open up again, rather than close.

I did everything I could to allow love in. I took care of myself through healthy nutrition, exercise, and meditation. I worked with a healer and coach to deal with my deep-seated negative beliefs and emotions. I spent time in nature and with friends to be reminded of what it felt like to belong. In the process of mending my "broken heart," my physical health improved. My resting heart rate became that of an elite athlete (in the low 50s, from the high 60s), and my "good" cholesterol, or HDL, jumped from 65 to 103.

Mimi Guarneri, a practicing cardiologist and author of *The Heart Speaks*, says that loneliness, anger, and grief can break hearts as easily as high blood pressure. She writes:

> *No one spoke of the other layers of the heart that didn't appear on a stress test or electrocardiogram, that are not taught in medical school: the mental heart, affected by hostility, stress and depression, . . . the emotional heart, able to be crushed by loss and grief, . . . the intelligent heart, with a nervous system all its own, . . . the spiritual heart, which yearns for a higher purpose, . . . and the universal heart, which communicates with others.*[1]

Your heart beats about 100,000 times in one day at an average of 80 beats per minute. It works even when you are at rest and pumps almost 2,000 gallons of blood per day through about 60,000 miles of blood vessels.[2] It delivers oxygen and nutrients, acts as a vehicle for chemical messengers like hormones, and removes waste products like carbon dioxide. It also acts like a "little brain," as it feels and picks up the subtlest of changes or threats to your body's state of balance and then communicates the information to your brain and other parts of your body.

Dr. J. Andrew Armour introduced the concept of a functional "heart brain" in 1991. In his work he showed that the heart has its own complex nervous system made up of a network of different types of neurons, neurotransmitters, proteins, and support cells like those found in the actual brain. This nerve circuitry, he found, enables the heart to act independently of the brain, to learn, remember, feel, and sense.[3]

You see, you have a magnificent, intelligent, powerful, yet also vulnerable heart that can teach you a lot about yourself and your world. It can feel imbalances in your environment, including changes in your emotions. It tells you when you are hurting and when you are well. It tells you when you are in harmony and when you are in disharmony. When you do not care for your heart, the disharmony can turn into dis-ease, though, especially if you have a genetic predisposition for heart disease. When you do care for your heart, it is often possible to move beyond genetic tendencies and ignite the power of your heart on every level—physically, emotionally, and spiritually—as you:

- Press the PAUSE button and become acquainted with the anatomy and functions of the cardiovascular system.

- OPTIMIZE your awareness of what can go wrong with the cardiovascular system, the signs and symptoms to watch out for that tell you to get medical help, and what you can learn from wisdom traditions and their view of the heart and its functions.

- Discover how your heart may be speaking to you as you WITNESS your physiology through guided exercises.

- EXAMINE the emotions and beliefs that your heart is holding on to that may be weakening your heart health.

- Develop the tools that will help you RELEASE negative habits and beliefs that are taxing your heart, RELIEVE your heart of its stress and worries, and RESTORE your heart's vitality.

PAUSE and OPTIMIZE Your Awareness of Your Heart

Anatomy and Functions

As you begin to learn about the heart and the circulatory system and its functions, keep in mind the notion that the heart's purpose is to pump the life force through you and help you ride through the ups and downs of life. For instance, it literally slows down when it is time for you to sleep and revs up when it is time for you to get up and get going. The heart's anatomy is built in such a way as to allow for such opposite functions to occur, so that you can stay flexible and adapt to change. For example, the heart pumps and contracts with a lot of force, yet it can also become very pliant and relaxed to allow the blood to flow in. It opens and closes, gives and receives, takes in and lets go. Your heart harmonizes opposite functions.

The heart has four chambers that are surrounded by thick, strong muscular walls, walls that can stay elastic and withstand pumping large volumes of blood out to the body with incredible force. These four chambers are the upper and lower sections and the right and left sides. The upper chambers are the right and left atria, and the lower chambers, the right and left ventricles. The walls of the left ventricle are the strongest and thickest, as this ventricle has to pump the blood the farthest, to the rest of the body, while the right ventricle only has to get the blood to the lungs. The heart chambers *force and relax, force and relax.*

Valves and walls, called septae, separate the chambers from one another. The atria are divided by the interatrial septum and the ventricles by the interventricular septum. The tricuspid valve, which has three leaflets, separates the right atrium from the right ventricle, and the mitral valve, which has two leaflets, separates the left atrium from the left ventricle. There is another valve between the right ventricle and the pulmonary artery called the pulmonic valve, as well as a valve between the left ventricle and the aorta, called the aortic valve. The purpose of the valves is to help keep the blood flowing forward and prevent backflow. The rhythm of the valves and septae is *open, then close, open, then close.*

Blood from the veins flows into the right atrium and then into the right ventricle. The right ventricle then pumps the blood to the pulmo-

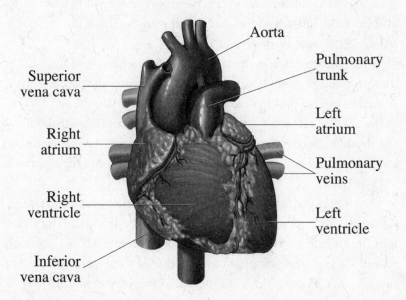

nary artery. The pulmonary artery splits into right and left to deliver the blood to each lung, where oxygen is put in and carbon dioxide is taken out. Oxygen-rich blood is then delivered back to the heart via the pulmonary vein. The blood moves from the left atrium to the left ventricle and is then pumped to the aorta, the largest artery of the heart. The aorta curves up and above the left ventricle, then turns down in front of the spinal cord to the abdomen. The rest of the arteries that deliver oxygen to other cells and organs branch off of the aorta, dividing into the smaller arterioles and into capillaries in the rest of the body, where oxygen and other nutrients are delivered to the organs and carbon dioxide and other waste products are removed.

Deoxygenated blood is then carried through small venules to larger veins, then to the inferior and superior vena cavae (the largest veins in the body), and then back to the heart. Waste products are eventually removed by the kidneys, liver, or lungs. Hormones, your body's chemical messengers, are also transported in the blood, acting as messengers that carry information and instruction from one organ to another, to and from the heart, and to and from the brain. The action here is *a taking in and then a letting go.*

A complex electrical system works to keep the heart beating at a regular pace and rhythm. Located in the right atrium, the pacemaker, or sinoatrial node, sends out electrical signals to initiate the contraction of the heart to set the rate, so that the rest of the heart can then follow the rhythm. Electrical pulses start in the atria and pass through the atrioventricular node, which then sends the pulses into the right and left ventricles.

In the first phase of the heartbeat, the ventricles are contracting, sending the blood to the lungs and into the body's circulatory system. This is called systole, the top number you see on a blood-pressure reading. The sound you might hear is caused by the valves between the atria and the ventricles closing to ensure there is no backflow of blood. In the second phase, the ventricles relax to allow the blood to flow in. This is called diastole, the bottom number you see on a blood-pressure reading. The heartbeat signals *movement,* which is then followed by *rest.*

I hope you are starting to get a clearer picture of the heart and how it works, enough to understand that its opposite functions enable you to maneuver and adapt to life's changes and challenges. These include force and relaxation, opening and closing, taking in and letting go, and regulating rest and activity. Imagine, if you will, that your heart got stiff and lost its ability to relax and stay pliant. It is not much different than when your body's muscles get tense. How flexible are you? How easy is it for you to get up and go?

Heart Dis-harmony and Dis-ease

The problem: too much force or too much relaxation. If the heart has to work too hard to force blood out, the muscles of the heart can become too thick or even too thin, a diseased state called a cardiomyopathy. If the heart muscles are too thick, or hypertrophic, they still may be able to force the blood out well, but their stiffness makes them unable to fully receive, expand, and fill with blood. When the walls are too thin or dilated, the walls can take the blood in, but can't force it out.

The problem: too open or too closed. The heart may also develop problems with its opening and closing capabilities, as infection, tumors, or plaque damages the valves and adjoining heart muscles. When the valves or septae are weak or malfunctioning, the result is backflow of blood. If the blood isn't moving forward, it is causing turbulence. Turbulence makes you more prone to blood clots. Blood clots can then create all kinds of havoc, as they travel through the circulatory system to other parts of the body, blocking blood vessels and blood flow, as we see in some cases of stroke.

Heart Dis-harmony and Dis-ease Facts

- By 2005, the total number of cardiovascular-disease deaths (mainly from coronary heart disease, stroke, and rheumatic heart disease) had increased globally from 14.4 million in 1990 to 17.5 million.

- Of these, 7.6 million were attributed to coronary heart disease and 5.7 million to stroke.

- The World Health Organization (WHO) estimates there will be about 20 million cardiovascular-disease deaths in 2015, accounting for 30 percent of all deaths worldwide.

- Cardiovascular-disease death is today the largest single contributor to global mortality and will continue to dominate mortality trends in the future.[4]

The problem: a blockage preventing giving and receiving. The flow of blood and therefore the flow of life can also be disturbed by the buildup of other substances, not just clots, like the fat buildup caused by high-fat diets and high cholesterol. These fatty plaques, also called atherosclerotic plaques, can cause the muscles or walls of the blood vessels to become thick and stiff, leading to poor blood flow or poor circulation. Poor circulation means less oxygen delivery and waste clearance, leading to more damage of the heart and other body tissues. When the blood vessels of the heart are damaged and provide poor oxygenation to the heart, it is known as coronary artery disease.

The problem: too slow (rest) or too fast (movement). The electrical circuitry of the heart is also susceptible to problems, causing the rhythm of the heartbeat to become irregular, also known as an arrhythmia.

The result of heart disharmony can be devastating. When blood flow and oxygen supply are impeded because of blood clots or the buildup of plaques, the heart cells scream for help, as oxygen supply becomes limited and they begin to die (called ischemia). An infarction means the cells have died, and the life force of the heart has now been really compromised. This is what happens when one experiences a "heart attack."

Red Flags That Tell You to Seek Help

Because of the high prevalence of heart disease, it is important for you to pay attention to any signs or symptoms your heart may be presenting to indicate you need medical attention. Know that your odds of surviving a heart attack improve if you seek attention within the first few hours of experiencing pain. Remember, the point of listing the red flags and warning signs is not to scare you, but to remind you that you have access to medical care that can help you. I also want to stress that learning about signs and symptoms will enable you to describe what it is you are feeling at any particular time, so that others, especially a qualified provider, can better diagnose what is going on and assist you.

For example, my dad has a long-standing history of heart disease. He is also not the best at providing his history and describing his symptoms. He tends to be stoic, says, "I'm fine," and then pushes himself, so that on a few occasions we have found him on the floor, looking pale and really not so "fine." After reading him the riot act several times, urging him to tell someone that he wasn't feeling well and to describe exactly what he was experiencing, my father finally did call me and his doctor one morning. He was able to describe his symptoms, which enabled us to better diagnose and help him, so that he would not end up in the emergency room with another cardiac event.

It really is understandable to want to avoid your symptoms, especially when your fear of what could be going on is so high. Our tendency often is to ignore whatever is wrong and hope it will go away. But as you are learning, it is never a good idea to ignore the body when it is speaking to you, as whispers will eventually become screams, especially when it concerns your heart.

If you are experiencing any of these symptoms, call 911 and take an aspirin (unless you are allergic).

CHEST PAIN: Men are more likely to experience chest pain when having a heart attack than women. Usually, the pain is described as crushing or like "an elephant sitting on one's chest." It can also present as a mild pain, more like a pressure in the breastbone, upper back, neck, or jaw, especially for women. The pain may start in the chest and radiate down the arm, to the back, jaw, or neck and may be associated with numbness.

Note that certain types of chest pain are *less likely* to be of cardiac origin. These include:

Pain that increases with a deep breath or when coughing

Pain that you can pinpoint with a finger

Pain that increases with pressure on the area

Pain that is constant (doesn't come and go), lasting hours or days

Pain that spreads to your legs

My patient Elisa's chest pain was so severe that she went to the emergency room. While there, waiting to be evaluated, she called me, and I asked her to describe her symptoms. She complained of an ache under her left breast that had been present constantly for four days and had gotten worse. She complained of shortness of breath with exertion, feeling very fatigued, but without any fever. Her pain was localized in that one spot and did not travel anywhere, but it did get worse when she took a deep breath. Elisa was only twenty-nine years old and had no family history of heart disease. I knew from Elisa's description that her symptoms were unlikely to be of cardiac origin, but it was good that she was getting evaluated. I suspected she had pneumonia, and a chest X-ray confirmed that.

FATIGUE: Since Elisa's symptoms were constant and were localized to one spot that she could pinpoint, I knew to look for causes other than heart. Elisa did the right thing by going to get evaluated and not being her own doctor, especially because she was feeling such extreme fatigue, another symptom to watch out for. Women especially are more prone to having fatigue or flulike symptoms without any chest pain when having a cardiac event.

OTHER SYMPTOMS: *Nausea* or *indigestion,* the latter of which can be a version of chest pain, may also occur, as well as *dizziness, fainting, shortness of breath, drenching sweats,* or *a sudden change in sleep patterns,* like a sudden awakening in the middle of the night. Some people experience a feeling of "impending doom" and unexplained *anxiety.* Though this may be a panic attack without a cardiac origin, I do recommend seeking medical attention immediately, especially if you have a personal or family history of cardiac problems.

SYMPTOMS THAT GET WORSE OVER TIME: When you experience any or all of these symptoms all of a sudden, you do want to seek attention right away. Often, though, you may experience all of the above symptoms, but to a lesser extent, perhaps over weeks or months. For instance, you may experience chest pain, shortness of breath, or nausea when you are really exerting yourself. Other signs and symptoms that could indicate there is a malfunction with your cardiovascular system include hair loss, erectile dysfunction, irregular heartbeat or palpitations, swollen feet or ankles, a dry or persistent cough, and pain, weakness, or coldness in your arms or legs. Do not put off seeking medical attention, even if the symptoms do not "seem that bad."

I will guide you to incorporate tools and techniques that can make your heart stronger and healthier, but there is no guarantee that these alone can fix an injured heart. Medications and interventions can get the cardiac system onto a better homeostatic baseline, so that the lifestyle and emotional changes you implement will have a better effect and will also allow you to someday get off the medication. *This is good news,* as the majority of problems can be prevented and heart harmony can be reinstilled by lifestyle changes and a reduction of risk factors.

Knowing Your Risk Factors

Some risk factors you can do nothing about, like getting older, having a first-degree relative who has heart disease or has had a stroke (before the age of fifty-five for a male relative or sixty-five for a female relative), being a man, being a postmenopausal woman (versus a premenopausal woman), and being of African or Asian descent. Having an autoimmune disease like lupus or rheumatoid arthritis may also put you at increased risk, but since lifestyle changes can offset the activity of inflammation, even this risk factor may be modified.[5]

These are the risk factors you have the ability to *influence:*

- A diet high in saturated fat is estimated to cause 31 percent of heart disease worldwide.

- Other conditions, such as high blood pressure, obesity, adult-onset diabetes, and high cholesterol (including high total cholesterol, triglycerides, and low-density lipoprotein, LDL, or low levels of high-density lipoprotein, HDL), increase your risks.

- Lack of physical activity increases your risk by 50 percent.

- Smoking or chewing tobacco increases your risk, especially if you started at a young age or are female.

- Drinking more than two alcoholic drinks a day may damage the heart muscle.

- A chronically stressful life, social isolation, anxiety, and depression increase your risk.[6]

You can especially address this last risk factor by looking to the medicine of wisdom traditions.

Wisdom Traditions and Heart Harmony

Wisdom traditions share the belief that the heart is the seat of our intelligence and our ability to love, communicate, heal, and maintain balance and harmony. It is believed that the heart works directly with the mind to guide us and our body to use our higher consciousness, sensations, and feelings to manage through the shifts and challenges we experience in our lives.

The heart is said to bring us into "oneness" with all of life, with the love that aligns us to all things and all beings and enables us to find harmony in opposites. When the heart is "open," we are more easily able to adapt to life's changes, doing so with optimism and inner tranquility. We can be forceful, yet relaxed, open to both giving and receiving, and able to know when we need to move and when we need to rest.

When the heart is "closed," wisdom traditions say, communication between the heart and mind are out of balance, so that there is a discrepancy between what we are feeling and what we are thinking. We may find we are more vulnerable to feeling emotional pain, hurt, anger, or envy. We are not in tune with the love and harmony within our own heart, which translates into a lack of harmony and rhythm in our life. As our heart shuts down, we may feel unable to move through life or find ourselves unable to be still. As our heart closes down, we may experience heart pain; mental confusion, as we cannot take in more information; or difficulty breathing, as we cannot fully take in deep breaths.

In all wisdom traditions, the key to a vibrant and healthy life is keeping the heart "open" to love and staying connected to others, one's spirit or soul, and the wonders or source of the universe, which some refer to as God, the Divine, or the Source. As love fills our hearts, we become stronger in mind and body, as the life force can now flow through our vessels and our hearts, which are open to connect to the infinite possibilities of life. Interestingly, today's science is finding that love and social bonds help us stay healthy and live longer and that love and deep connections are the way to have a fulfilled life.[7]

As you learn more about how to POWER up your heart, you therefore want to keep in mind the theme of harmony, asking yourself such questions as:

How well do I both give and receive?

How well do I manage my energy? Do I give myself time to rest, so that I can move forward full force?

How open or closed am I to new ideas, people, or experiences?

Do I trust love?

Do I share my thoughts and ideas with others, or do I tend to keep things to myself?

Do I have a tendency to feel connected or disconnected to others or the world around me?

One day I was in session with a patient, Elaine.

"How do I make the pain go away?" Elaine asked.

"What pain?" I asked.

"The pain I feel in my heart every time my family argues or my children yell at me. I am anxious often, and I get very upset when there are disagreements in the family. The last time it happened, I had severe chest pain and I went to the emergency room. My blood pressure was really high, but there were no EKG changes, and they found no other problems with my heart. They told me it was stress and to follow up with my doctor. I take Ativan for the anxiety when I need to, but it doesn't make the pain go away completely, and I don't like to take it because it makes me woozy."

"I do understand why you would be upset when there are family arguments. But why do you think you also feel so much anxiety? Has anything really bad ever happened to you, your family, or someone you love?"

Elaine thought about the question for a bit and answered, "Now that I think about it, I am not so sure. I don't like fighting or discordance, but I am not sure why it makes me so anxious, especially when nothing bad has happened. It usually ends with apologies and a big dinner."

"Why don't we ask your heart," I said.

Elaine then closed her eyes, took several deep breaths to clear her mind, and then directed her focus to her heart. She allowed herself to revisit an experience when the family had argued, and she immediately noted a squeezing sensation in her chest. I asked Elaine to ask her heart why it was creating such a sensation and to guide her to a memory that would help her understand.

Then Elaine said, "I am seeing myself at seven years old. My mom had just died from leukemia. Dad couldn't take care of me on his own, so we moved in with his sister. My dad didn't know what to do with me, so most of the time he would keep busy at work, and when he was

home, he would spoil me with presents. My aunt's children were jeal-
ous, and I guess maybe my aunt resented me. She yelled at me a lot. The
other kids yelled at me too. I tried to be a good girl. I really missed my
mother. I still do."

Elaine began to cry. She cried because she had missed out on having
an experience of being in a happy family and, most of all, because she
lost her mom when she was so young.

"It happened so long ago. I cannot believe I still carry this pain
around. I went to therapy for twenty-five years. I thought I had dealt
with this story."

"I am not sure the pain ever fully goes away," I answered. "Losing
someone is painful, especially when you are so young and cannot fully
understand why. Perhaps your undeveloped mind associated the pain of
losing your mom with a family that fights, so when your family argues,
it causes the pain to come back. We cannot know for sure, but we can try
to heal the pain from your loss and see what happens. Also, if your life
is not filled with other joys, love, or appreciation, especially for yourself,
this hurt can take up a lot of space, which can lead to your perception of
experiencing a lot of pain with the slightest provocation. When you fill
your life with good—love, laughter, friends, beauty, nature, and so on—
your heart can expand so that, relatively speaking, the pain in your heart
is smaller. In other words, your hurt is not really smaller, but relative to
the rest of the heart, it is taking up less space, so you feel it less. The pain
doesn't go away, necessarily; your heart is simply large enough to hold it."

Over the course of several months, Elaine worked on incorporating
more joy, love, and nature in her life. She learned to practice mindfulness, to be able to stay present in the moment with appreciation and
grace. She also learned meditation practices that allowed her to release
the pain of loss and fill her heart with love and compassion instead.
Over time, Elaine discovered that she had the capacity to be more loving and present with people and be able to truly appreciate the gifts in

her life. She discovered that taking care of her health was not just about exercise and eating healthy, but also healing her heart.

Elaine learned the meaning of keeping an open heart. She came to notice that when she felt separate, disconnected, and fearful, she would experience tension in her chest that signified that her heart was "closed." At these times, she noted, her blood pressure would go up too. When she felt joyful, connected, and hopeful, in contrast, she experienced an incredible capacity to breathe more fully and deeply and the sensation that her heart was more "open." Elaine also found that her blood pressure was always stable during these times.

Wisdom Traditions and Science Merge

If you were to think about the first time your heart was broken, do you also notice a little twinge in your chest? Why is it that your heart still "hurts" when it happened so long ago?

Although you can use reason to overcome a trauma to a certain degree, your emotions and beliefs related to the event may still be so strong that your emotional memory triggers the stress response. That stress response involves an increase in stress hormones and changes in the cardiovascular system. The resulting change—whether it is a contraction of the heart muscles or the blood vessels or a speeding up of the heart—is often palpable.

Interestingly, you don't always have to be consciously aware of a negative situation or memory for this reaction to occur. Your heart may be able to sense that something is wrong in your environment before your mind registers it. For example, you might find you can feel "tension" in a room without knowing the reason.

Though wisdom traditions have been alluding to the heart's power to feel and to "know" for thousands of years, scientists today are finding out why this might be true. According to the director of research at the

Institute of HeartMath, Rollin McCraty, "The heart generates the largest electromagnetic field in the body. The electrical field as measured in an electrocardiogram (ECG) is about 60 times greater in amplitude than the brain waves recorded in an electroencephalogram (EEG)."[8]

With its large electromagnetic field, it seems the heart can sense danger before your brain does; the stress response is activated physiologically way before your executive functioning brain might comprehend why. Your heart will also sense when you are safe and feeling loved, which your mind may register as just a sense of ease. For example, you might simply feel uncomfortable around a certain person, though you do not know why; the person seems perfectly nice, and a week earlier you really enjoyed spending time together. Later you find out this individual was extremely anxious about getting a test result.

Why does this happen? How does the heart know how to "pick up the energy" of another person? Modern science is still looking into this query, but what we do know is that your memories, thoughts, beliefs, and emotions affect the internal environment of your body, and this includes your heart. And given that the heart has very complex neural wiring, its electromagnetic field can likely pick up more subtle sensations and vibrational changes, like the change in the beat of music. One theory is that the change or sensation sends a signal to the heart, which then connects that signal with an emotional memory (positive or negative), which results in a physiological response.

What do I mean by emotional memory? Let's say deep within your memory lies an experience when you were hurt or betrayed in a relationship long ago. You have gone through therapy, and you believe you are completely healed. The problem is that every time you go out on a date, you get palpitations. You may shrug it off to just being nervous about dating, which may be true, but it may also be that you still carry underlying fears associating love with betrayal.

You can't know until you ask your heart.

WITNESS the Physiology of Your Heart

For starters, you want to notice how your heart responds to positive or negative imagery or thoughts. You want to notice what it feels like when it is "open" and when it is "closed."

AWARENESS EXERCISE

Close your eyes, and begin with the practice of emptying the mind.

Then bring your awareness to your chest, to your heart, and notice what your chest feels like. As the breath moves in and out, does the chest feel open or closed, relaxed or tight, heavy or light, and if so where?

Simply acknowledge your heart and notice.

Acknowledge that your heart carries all your memories, from the past and the present. Notice.

Introduce yourself, and see if the heart answers back. Open, closed, relaxed, tight, heavy or light? Where? Notice.

What happens with your breath?

Do not rush this exercise. Give yourself time to identify your feelings and bodily sensations accompanying each of these words or images:

Sad

Joyful

Not enough time

Plenty of time

Open

Closed

I am bad

I am good

White sandy beach

Garbage dump

Injustice

Triumph

The face of someone who angers you or someone you dislike

The face of someone you love

Notice what you feel or sense. Notice associated emotions. Does your chest open or close, feel relaxed or tight, heavy or light, and if so, where?

You may note that joyful or positive words or images elicit a relaxed feeling in your chest and a more positive attitude or state of mind. The opposite happens with more negative or upsetting words or examples. For instance, looking at a garbage dump might lead you to feel less enthusiastic about what tomorrow will bring than if you were looking at a sunset.

Which word or image caused you to have the strongest reaction? Why would this be? Ready to find out?

EXAMINE Your Deeper Emotions and Beliefs

GOING DEEPER EXERCISE

Empty your mind as you breathe in deeply and exhale slowly and completely.

Bring your awareness to your chest again.

Notice your breath moving in and out.

Ask your heart to explain to you why it closed or became tight or constricted from one or more of the above words or images.

Perhaps you can ask your heart to show you a story from your past associated with the feeling. Maybe it was a time you felt disappointed, betrayed, or hurt.

Ask the heart to show you the imagery, the words, or the experience associated with this feeling.

Then ask your heart one or more of the following questions:

How does this situation make me feel about being loved or valued?

Did I feel safe to express myself in this situation, or do I feel safe today in ones like it? If not, why not?

Why am I scared to fully open my heart? What may happen? Why am I holding back?

Do I become more rigid in my ways when I feel this way? How do I act toward myself, loving or destructive?

When I feel this way, do I tend to force my opinions on others by being defensive or argumentative, or can I take in other people's opinions in a relaxed way?

How flexible am I when I feel this way? Am I capable of both giving and receiving, or I do more of one than the other?

What anger or negativity am I still holding on to in my heart and why?

When I feel this way, do I feel more anxious or calm? Do I need to sit still or sleep or keep moving?

Notice what you see, hear, sense or feel. Take your time to allow thoughts and answers to come forward.

When you are ready, pick up your pen and paper and write about your experience, thoughts, and feelings. See if you can uncover the underlying belief behind this memory and what it is you really need. As you write, look for a prominent pattern or story that often appears in your life experiences. Can you accept and be accountable for your role of upholding this story?

RELEASE, RELIEVE, and RESTORE

After you have completed the examination of your heart, you may be ready to release what you have uncovered and choose to work on living with an open heart, as you also incorporate the lifestyle changes and activities that enable you to truly be healthy and happy. The goal is for you to relieve yourself of the stressors and strains, then reward your heart and restore harmony to it.

This means learning to let go of toxins and waste products that include negative emotions, thoughts, and memories; allow in only that which nurtures you. It means understanding the importance of being active, yet also resting, giving and also receiving, and staying open rather than being closed to love and life's possibilities. By creating harmony in opposites in your life, in other words, you help your heart get healthy.

Letting Go of the Bad, Taking In the Good

You are now ready to examine the growth that came out of the negative thoughts or experiences you uncovered. Elaine, for instance, was able to see what an incredibly loving family she had created in spite of her childhood experience. You want to look at what abilities, positive qualities, or gifts you acquired as a direct or indirect result of a past experience. Here, you may choose to write about your three "Vs": virtues, values, and victories. Elaine was able to see that she was a strong, kind, and compassionate person who had strong family values and who indeed did create the strong and loving family that she so appreciated.

Now, choose a virtue, value, or victory and then do the following exercise.

Is this story even true?

Is it true that _____ (fill in)?

What are the positive takeaways from this memory?

What is positive about me? What are my virtues, victories, and values?

When you have come up with your three "Vs," choose one that resonates most deeply and positively with you and do the following:

OPENING THE HEART MEDITATION

Empty your mind, inhaling as you count to three, exhaling as you count to five.

Keep the same rhythm of the breath and focus on your heart.

As you exhale, imagine you are letting go of the negative memory and all the feelings and beliefs that go along with it. Do this for at least five breath cycles.

As you inhale, imagine you are filling your heart with infinite love and compassion that come from the surrounding universe. Do this at for at least five breath cycles.

On the sixth cycle, imagine your heart is free and can now bloom like a flower.

Say these words as often as you wish: "I like the feeling of _____" (fill in your chosen virtue, value, or victory).

Notice how you feel and when or if you want to, write about the experience and your intention to remember to feel this way anytime your specific negative feeling, memory, or sensation arises.

SMOKING: If you smoke, now is the time to stop. It is never too late! I know it is an addiction that is not easy to give up, and I won't go into the reasons or the venues to do so. Do ask yourself though if you love yourself enough to live life fully and completely without numbing your feelings. Addictions are really habits that started as a way to cope. Perhaps when you instill new and healthy coping tools, you won't need to smoke. You may want to do the Witnessing or Examining Exercise on the issue of why you smoke, what need it fulfills, and how it makes you feel. You can then use this book to help you find new outlets of relief that enable you feel calm and relaxed—maybe even more so than with nicotine.

OTHER MEDICAL PROBLEMS: If you have high blood pressure or any other forms of heart disease, do see your doctor and take your medications. As you develop better lifestyle habits, including a meditation practice, you may very well be able to get off the medications or at least lower the dosages. Until you have built up your tools though, you want to keep your heart and blood vessels in as much homeostatic balance as possible.

The same goes if you are diabetic. Hemodynamic or blood-sugar instability presents a big stress on the body, which means more stress response reactivity and a higher allostatic load on your heart. It is absolutely possible, in many cases, to work closely with your doctor to wean yourself off medications as you create other outlets of relief that enable your body to be in homeostatic balance.

If you have high cholesterol, you may be able to keep it down with a healthy diet and exercise routine. If you are at high risk for heart disease, please check with your doctor, as medications are recommended to keep your LDL below a certain level.

Finally, studies are now connecting some instances of heart disease with poor dental hygiene.[9] Follow healthy dental hygiene practices and follow up with your dentist for regular teeth cleaning.

Regulating Rest and Movement

MOVING YOUR BODY: Your heart needs movement. Exercise helps keep your blood pressure, blood sugar, and cholesterol down, while helping your mood stay up. If you do have heart disease, check with your doctor to see what sort of exercise restrictions you may have. In general, you want to always choose an activity that you enjoy and that you are most likely to do. Your goal is to accomplish about two and a half hours of moderate exercise (you can have a conversation) or seventy-five minutes of vigorous exercise (conversation is not possible) per week. Moderate exercise can include brisk walking for twenty-plus minutes a day. If you do it out in nature, you will likely keep going and not notice that you are tired. If you like running, swimming, cycling, or interval training, you really just need about fifteen minutes a day of such vigorous aerobic activity or twenty-five minutes three times a week.[10] I always find that exercise is more likely to happen if you have a buddy, so rally some of your friends to get fit with you, or join a walking, biking, running, dancing, or other group exercise that suits you.

If you are usually a couch potato, start slowly and do something fun. Park your car farther from the store, so that you have to walk more. Turn on the music and dance.

LOVING LIFESTYLE CHOICES: The heart enjoys being nurtured. You can do so by ensuring you give it time to rest. Get adequate sleep, and even consider a regular meditation practice, which will bring your stress response down, along with adrenalin and cortisol levels. Taking breaks throughout the day to walk out in nature, do some deep breathing, or socialize with a friend all a happy heart doth make. You need *quiet* time in your very busy life to rest and recondition your heart. Remember the cycle of the heart is to get up and go *and* rest. If you are having a hard time resting, consider getting a massage or some form of relaxing bodywork during which the gentle touch can soothe you into resting.

You may also develop a meditation practice of some sort, as there is increasingly more evidence pointing to the benefits of relaxation techniques for cardiovascular health.[11] You can choose to do the above Opening the Heart Meditation as a daily practice.

Eating to Fuel and Perform

There are a multitude of resources for you on bookshelves and online that offer guides to following a nutrition plan that can boost your heart health. As you learned in the previous chapter, you want to work on avoiding foods that can tax your system and increase inflammation. In this section, I want to concentrate on what you want to eat to power your heart. The key is to enjoy yourself, but to also remember that food is the *fuel* that enables you to perform functions from lifting heavy weights and fighting infection to getting through a stressful day. Try to focus on this notion rather than on food as a way to relieve your stress.

There are definitely food groups that can boost your heart health. The following are the common questions my patients ask and what I tell them (you can visit the NIH website, www.nhlbi.nih.gov, for more information on recipes for a healthy heart[12]):

What fats are good for my heart?

Fatty acids like omega-3 fatty acids—as I mentioned, found in fatty fish like salmon and tuna and nuts like almonds—and alpha-linolenic acid—found in plant foods like Brussels sprouts, kale, spinach and salad greens, ground flaxseed, and walnuts— help lower inflammation, reduce blood clots, and protect against heart disease and can increase your good cholesterol, or HDL, levels. If you cannot get enough omega-3 in your diet, you can choose to take a supplement, though you want to check with your doctor for the best dosage for you, especially if you are already on a blood thinner.

I heard that nuts and seeds are good for me. Is that true?

Nuts like almonds and walnuts are high in omega-3 fatty acids and also offer phytosterols, minerals (like magnesium), and other vitamins (like vitamins E and C), which can act as antioxidants, protecting your heart cells from oxidative stress damage, as I discussed in the previous chapter.

I know fruits and vegetables are good for my heart, but which ones and why?

Surprise, surprise—dark leafy greens help your heart stay healthy. As you have also learned in the previous chapter, greens provide you with a multitude of vitamins, minerals, and anti-oxidants (like polyphenols). Spinach, bell peppers, asparagus, and broccoli, for example, are loaded with carotenoids, a heart-protective antioxidant. Vegetables like spinach and asparagus are also a great source for folic acid and B-complex vitamins (like B12 and B6), which can help protect against clots and hardening of the arteries. B3, also called niacin, can help lower your bad cholesterol, or LDL.

Blueberries and many other berries, dark plums, dark grapes (the reason red wine is so good for you!), and apples are a great source of polyphenols, antioxidants that protect blood vessels, lower blood pressure, and lower LDL. Other fruits such as cantaloupe, for instance, give you antioxidants like carotenoids and vitamin C as well as potassium. Potassium is crucial for powering your heart function, as it promotes good muscle contraction and transmission of nerve impulses.

What about grains? Which ones are good for my heart?

A variety of grains offer the needed vitamins, minerals, and antioxidants, like brown rice, which is a great source of B vitamins, or oatmeal, a great source of omega-3 fatty acids and heart-healthy fiber.

Something to keep in mind when you are adding starches to your diet is that you want to choose those that are low on the glycemic index. The glycemic index is a measure of how foods affect your blood-sugar levels. If a food group has a high glycemic index, it means it is absorbed quickly, so that your blood-sugar levels spike, followed by a fast rise in insulin. Higher insulin levels are associated with more inflammation and other diseases, including heart disease. Foods high on the glycemic index include natural sugar, syrups, and fruit juices, not just cookies and chocolate cake.

Foods that are low on the glycemic index, in contrast, are absorbed more slowly and allow for milder release of insulin without the associated inflammatory response. Because some grains can be fairly high on the glycemic index, I generally recommend keeping your daily grain intake to no larger than the palm of your hand and focusing on getting most of your carbohydrates from plants and fruits. Two of my favorite carbohydrate sources are sweet potatoes and yams, which are good sources of carotenoids, vitamins, and fiber.

Learning to Give and Receive, Staying Open and Not Closed

CONNECTING WITH OTHERS: Studies have shown an association between heart disease and a lack of social support or social isolation.[13] We certainly know that social support plays an important role in how you react and handle stress, which may be one explanation for why folks do better when they have love and support. A study of forty-six patients who had suffered a severe stroke, for instance, showed that those individuals who had a good social support system scored 65 percent higher on mobility tests and their ability to perform daily tasks six months later. They also improved faster compared to those individuals who had less social support.[14]

Support comes in many forms. It enables you to feel less alone and overwhelmed and literally gives you the actual help you need. Support can be emotional, physical, mental, spiritual, or informational.

I am guessing many of you are good at offering help or an ear to listen, but not so great at receiving. Well, support has to be a two-way street. Work on receiving from friends or family. Join a group, perhaps a spiritual group or community, where you share like passions. Meet with a therapist or counselor if you want someone to talk to who can be objective. And last but not least, get or borrow a pet. There is nothing like the unconditional love you can get from your animals.

GRATITUDE, COMPASSION, AND GENEROSITY: Acts of gratitude, compassion, and generosity all stem from an open heart, from a mindset or belief that you have so much already, that you want to give and share. Studies in fact show that individuals who practice gratitude have stronger immune systems, more joy, and more positive emotions and attitudes and feel less lonely.[15] Science also shows that generosity, or helping others, buffers stress and lowers mortality.[16] It seems also that when you show more compassion, including to yourself, you just might live longer, as stress response reactivity and inflammation are lowered.

It doesn't take much to be generous or compassionate, and it certainly is quite easy to find snippets of gratitude in your life. It may mean slowing down a bit and taking the time to appreciate what you have, rather than what you don't. You can commit a random act of generosity—an extra dollar in your tip to the server; an extra minute or more to your colleague who has a problem that needs to be discussed; some room for your child to make a mistake; a smile to a stranger on the street.

Keep a *gratitude journal.* Every day, write three to five things you feel grateful for. Perhaps you feel lucky that you found a great parking spot. Perhaps you appreciate the beautiful blue sky, that you enjoyed the healthy food you put into your body, and that you were able to spend some time with someone you adore. As you accumulate your list, you may find you can step back and view events in your life with a different eye, perhaps see the blessings in disguise even in challenging situations.

Try waking up every morning ready to *savor* the day. Tell yourself that you are so looking forward to having another beautiful day! From the minute you open your eyes and begin the activities of your day, savor each moment. Notice beauty. Notice tastes. For instance, perhaps you find yourself feeling frustrated at work. Taking a moment to remember how delicious your breakfast was will counteract the negative emotions and feelings and enable you to maintain a better outlook and perhaps even problem-solve better.

COMPASSION TOWARD YOURSELF: Most of us live in a constant state of comparing ourselves to others, to our own expectations, or to the expectations of others and labeling ourselves as either "good" or "bad." I encourage you now to throw away all labels and begin to simply appreciate and love yourself as who you are. In other words, practice self-compassion. Self-compassion enables individuals to accept who they are and to view their circumstances as manageable. Catch yourself when you put yourself or someone else down and instead remember you are a human being who is living, learning, and loving every day.

LAUGHTER: In my opinion, there is often no better remedy for maintaining a healthy heart than laughter and the ability to fully enjoy life. The research is inconclusive as to why laughter is so good for you. Some studies have pointed to blood cells becoming less sticky; others, to improvement in blood flow.[17] But you know what I say to that? Who cares? Laughter feels good, and it is usually social, so other people are feeling good with you. You can feel your own heart opening just by thinking of laughing. Try it—you might like it.

CHAPTER SIX

The Lungs

Letting In and Letting Go

Breath is the bridge which connects life to consciousness,
which unites your body to your thoughts. Whenever
your mind becomes scattered, use your breath
as the means to take hold of your mind again.

—THÍCH NHAT HAHN, *THE MIRACLE OF MINDFULNESS*

I t is believed by many wisdom traditions that breath is a metaphor for
life and breathing represents the essence of our being. The polarity of
the "in" and "out" of breath is likened to the polarity seen in nature,
such as night and day, the waves that roll in and out, and the flower that
blooms and withers to earth. Like the heart, the lungs find harmony in
opposite functions that maintain a continuous cycle of expansion and
contraction, taking in and letting go.

Have you tried to hold your breath recently? Try it. Of course, you
can't hold your breath for too long even if you try. Mechanisms in
your body and brain override any voluntary attempt you make at not

breathing. You can change the rhythm or pace, but you can't stop the breath. The cycle simply continues.

You breathe twelve to twenty-five breaths per minute without even knowing it. You can choose to breathe faster or slower, depending on your state of mind and conscious awareness. But other than that, you have little control over whether or not you breathe. What or who has control? The receptors in your blood vessels and your brain make the final decision, and the decision is based on your state of homeostasis, or balance.

Since your lungs are part of your first-line-of-defense team, helping you get rid of infection, foreign objects, and carbon dioxide, it is necessary that you have a sensory system that can tell your brain and your lungs when you need to cough, breathe faster, or breathe slower. Damage to your lungs or this sensory system can limit their ability to protect the body, clear it of toxins, and fill it with the good stuff, oxygen. When the lungs suffer, their ability to expand and contract, let in and let go, is impeded, which means your body is less capable of releasing toxins in exchange for oxygen, your source for energy, vitality, and ultimately power.

In this chapter, you will learn how to regain or enhance the POWER of your lungs as you:

- Press the PAUSE button and become acquainted with the anatomy and functions of your lungs.

- OPTIMIZE your awareness of how your lungs can become damaged or weak, the signs and symptoms that tell you to get medical help, and how the lungs are also portals to your vitality and well-being as explained by wisdom traditions.

- Discover how your lungs may be speaking to you as you WITNESS your physiology through guided exercises.

- EXAMINE emotions and beliefs related to letting go or to your sense of self that may be lying deep within your lungs.

- Develop the tools that will help you RELEASE old habits or beliefs that do not serve you, RELIEVE your lungs of stress and toxins, and RESTORE to your lungs their full breathing power.

PAUSE and OPTIMIZE Your Awareness of Your Lungs

Anatomy and Functions

You have two lungs, right and left, located in your chest cavity inside your rib cage. They are built to exchange gas between your blood and the air, taking oxygen in, letting carbon dioxide out, and keeping the pH, or acid, concentration regulated. In order to be able to expand and contract, the lungs are made up of spongy, elastic tissue. Did you know that if you were to stretch out the inner surface of the lungs it would take up about 50 to 70 square meters (538 to 753 square feet)?[1]

The lungs are surrounded by two membranes called pleura, an inside layer directly covering the outside surface of the lungs (visceral pleura) and an outside layer attached to the wall of the chest cavity (parietal pleura). In between the two pleura is a hollow space called the pleural cavity, which enables the lungs to expand when you inhale. It is in this space that the pleura secrete serous fluid to keep the lungs lubricated and protect them from getting inflamed or irritated.

When you inhale, air first enters your mouth or your nose, passes through the pharynx, larynx, and then the trachea. The trachea then splits into the right and left bronchi for each lung. Each bronchus is made up of smooth muscle and cartilage that form incomplete rings that look like Cs. The bronchus is lined with little hairs, or cilia, that sweep dust and pathogens away, and goblet cells, which secrete mucus that also sweeps the pathogens out.

In each lobe of each lung, the bronchi break up several more times into small bronchioles. Bronchioles contain elastin rather than cartilage, making them even more flexible and pliant, so that they can change in size depending on the body's requirements for oxygen. For instance, they expand during exercise and contract in a dust storm. Bronchioles divide further into terminal bronchioles, which bring the air to the alveoli, or air sacs. Gas exchange between the lungs and the blood occurs here, as the alveoli are each surrounded by many tiny capillaries in the interstitial space. As the air sacs are fragile, they also require lubrication or surfactant, provided by septal cells, as well as protection from pathogens, provided for by immune cells called macrophages.

Air will move from a high-pressure area to a lower one. When you inhale, the muscles between your ribs (intercostal muscles) and the diaphragm expand to create less pressure inside the chest cavity compared to the outside pressure. This allows the air to flow into the lungs and inflate them like a balloon. When the muscles and diaphragm relax, the volume inside the chest cavity gets smaller, resulting in a pressure buildup and forcing the air to flow out of the lungs to where the pressure is less.

As soon as the lungs have let go of the air, a new cycle of breath begins, without much thought on your part, because your lower brain and the autonomic nervous system are in charge. The nerve cells in the respiratory centers of your brain stem send out signals to the diaphragm and the intercostal muscles at regular intervals to relax and contract. These nerve cells can be influenced by signals coming in from other parts of your body. For instance, special nerve cells in the aorta and carotid arteries, called chemoreceptors, monitor the acid level (pH) and oxygen and carbon-dioxide concentrations in the blood and relay this information to the respiratory center in the brain. If the oxygen concentration is low, the carbon dioxide is high, or the pH is low (acidic), the respiratory centers will speed up your breathing rate, so that you blow out more carbon dioxide until the levels are normalized. Your lower brain (brain stem) has another chemoreceptor that monitors the carbon-dioxide levels in the cerebral spinal fluid.

Your higher brain, or your executive functioning mind, also has a say when it comes to your breathing. When you are in pain or are experiencing negative emotions, your hypothalamus will stimulate you to breathe faster. Other neurons in the cortex allow you to choose to hold your breath or speed up or slow down the rate of breathing.

Like the heart, the lungs also have nerve cells, or a "little brain," that monitors the local environment for changes. Nerve cells screen for unwanted particles and substances like smoke or dust and signal the respiratory center when to contract the diaphragm and respiratory muscles so that you will cough, which allows the air to violently and rapidly leave your lungs. Other nerve cells, or stretch receptors, monitor the expansion of your lungs. If your lungs expand too much, the receptors will signal the lungs to deflate.

It's a pretty amazing system, really. The problem is that it is also highly vulnerable to damage.

What Can Go Wrong

Your lungs are part of your first line of defense against toxins. This means the lungs get hit first, and often hit hard, making them more prone to damage or disease. If you are overexposed to irritants like smoke, for instance, your lungs can get inflamed or become exposed to oxidative stress, which, as you have learned, can result in a whole host of medical conditions.

To understand how problems can arise, I find it best to focus on the functions and how or where they can be weakened.

BLOCKED AIRWAYS: When airways are blocked, air can't go in and out. With asthma, the airways become inflamed, and they may spasm and narrow. Wheezing and shortness of breath ensue. Triggers include infections, pollution, allergies, extreme cold weather, and exercise. Another form of airway blockage occurs with the genetic condition cystic fibrosis, in which there is a problem with mucus clearing, so that individuals are more susceptible to lung infections, which can create more damage. A more chronic condition called chronic obstructive pulmonary disease (COPD) is a result of blockage of the airways that progresses over time. Chronic bronchitis or constant inflammation and mucus production as well as emphysema fall into this category, and tumors or cancer growths can also cause airway blockage.

DAMAGED ALVEOLI: Damage to the alveoli can cause inadequate exchange of gases. With emphysema, damage can be so widespread that not only are the airways affected, but also the little air sacs, or alveoli, where the gas exchange occurs (where carbon dioxide is exchanged for oxygen). Pneumonia or an infection due to bacteria, viruses, or fungi can also injure the alveoli, as can the fluid overload that happens with heart failure. The alveoli can also be hurt when exposed to trauma from the inhalation of certain substances like smoke, coal dust, or asbestos. Serious cases of pneumonia, smoke inhalation, or other illnesses can severely injure the alveoli, leading to acute respiratory distress syndrome (ARDS), a life-threatening problem requiring the person to receive mechanical ventilation to survive until recovery occurs. Cancer affecting the lungs can invade and harm the larger airways as well as the alveoli.

DAMAGED PLEURA: Damage to the pleura can cause loss of elasticity. For the lungs to let in and let go, they need to be able to fully expand and contract. The interstitial space and their elastic lining, or pleura, enable them to do just that. Both are susceptible to injury, however, which can result in rigidity or loss of elasticity of the lungs. Autoimmune disorders and conditions, like systemic lupus erythematosus and tuberculosis (respectively), for example, can lead to inflammation and damage that eventually lead to scarring, or fibrosis. The pleura can be damaged by the backflow of fluid from heart failure, pneumonia, inflammation, or trauma. Mesothelioma is a cancer of the pleura. It is usually associated with a prolonged exposure to asbestos.

For the purposes of this chapter, it is less important for you to know about the different lung conditions and more important that you understand the functions of the lungs, specifically where the problems might arise, so you are better suited to avoid risk factors.

Risk Factors

The American Lung Association Epidemiology and Statistics Unit monitors trends in lung disease and behavioral risk factors. They conduct analyses of raw data from government surveys and develop reports on lung disease, mortality, economic costs, prevalence, hospitalization, and risk factors.

There are many ways to protect your lungs and avoid the risk factors that may lead to such injuries or damage, so that you do not become one of these statistics. Of course, some risk factors are not modifiable, like genetics and age. For instance, you are more prone to lung infections as you get older, and there is a correlation between family history and lung cancers and some with asthma.[6] The extent to which genetic or inherited factors are involved, however, is really not fully understood.

What we do know is that there are many risk factors that can be avoided or corrected. For instance, active smoking is responsible for close to 90 percent of lung cancer cases, while 10 percent are due to radon exposure, and 1–2 percent due to air pollution.[7]

The Breathless Facts

- In a 2011 report, the American Lung Association found that 20.5 million adults in the United States had asthma, and that 14.7 million reported having COPD.[2]

- According to the Centers for Disease Control (CDC), more people die of lung cancer in the United States than of any other cancer.[3]

- In 2010 (the most recent year for which numbers are available), 201,144 people in the United States were diagnosed with lung cancer, 107,164 men and 93,980 women.[4]

- It appears that men develop lung cancer more often than women, according to a 2008 survey.[5]

When you smoke, you increase your risk for a multitude of lung problems including bronchitis, lung cancer, COPD, and emphysema. The more you smoke, the more likely you will have a problem, including an increased chance of getting lung cancer. Air pollution can increase lung problems such as asthma, bronchitis, and some lung cancers. For example, people who are exposed to a lot of diesel exhaust fumes, asbestos, uranium, and radon are at a higher risk of lung cancer. You are also more likely to develop asthma when chronically exposed to dust, molds, or certain chemicals.[8]

Red Flags That Your Lungs Need Medical Attention

Whatever the cause or risk factor may be, once the injury has occurred, your lungs will certainly give you a warning that you need to see a health-care professional. If you have ever experienced shortness of breath, you know it is one of the most scary and unpleasant occurrences. Since anxiety can make the symptoms worse, you want to try and remain calm and seek the help you need. An initial evaluation will likely include a measure of your oxygen level, a chest X-ray, or possibly a CT scan, MRI, or other type of radiographic test.

SHORTNESS OF BREATH: If you develop breathing problems like wheezing, or the shortness of breath is becoming progressively worse, you want to seek medical attention. This could be an experience of breathlessness or the feeling that you can't get enough air. The shortness of breath may also be accompanied by noise other than wheezing, like rattling or gurgling, which may indicate fluid accumulation or infection. If you cannot speak, speed dial 911 and get help quickly. If you do have asthma or COPD and your relief medicine is not working or you do not have access to any, go to the emergency room for treatment.

PERSISTENT COUGH: A persistent cough, a new cough, or a cough that won't go away or becomes worse needs to be evaluated by a doctor. Coughing up blood or mucus can occur with a variety of conditions, including bronchitis and lung cancer. If the cough is chronic, not going away, and accompanied by blood, you want to make sure you have an evaluation as soon as possible.

RECURRENT LUNG INFECTIONS: Having repeated lung infections, whether bronchitis or pneumonia, may be a warning that your immune system is suppressed, that you have a blockage caused by a tumor, or that there is another underlying condition that is disabling your lungs from clearing the disease. You need further evaluation by a physician.

PERSISTENT FATIGUE: Almost all lung conditions, because they affect your breathing and oxygen supply, can intermittently lead to feelings of fatigue. However, fatigue that is persistent or worsening may be a sign of an underlying condition such as cancer, heart disease, or anemia, and therefore requires an immediate evaluation.

UNEXPLAINED WEIGHT LOSS: Weight loss can also accompany many illnesses, including cancer. Usually, if the weight loss is more than 10 pounds and you cannot attribute the loss to less eating or more exercise, this warrants an evaluation.

OTHER SYMPTOMS: *Loss of appetite* can occur with any worsening of lung conditions, including COPD and cancer, as can *poor sleep* and early morning *headaches,* which indicate your oxygen supply is poor during sleep. Often, since many lung problems are either caused by or associated with heart issues, there may also be *swelling* of the ankles, legs, or abdomen.

In my clinical experience, most lung problems are treatable, especially when patients address their underlying spiritual or emotional beliefs and learn relaxation and breathing exercises. When patients resolve their negative attitudes toward letting go, the creation of loving boundaries and self-nurturance, and the need to be more expansive, their lung problems usually get better along the way.

The Lungs as Seen in Wisdom Traditions

Intrinsically, in most wisdom traditions, the lungs represent nature's way of cleansing and renewing. They function to enhance the life force;

as they expand, they bring the wonders and beauty of heaven and earth into our breath and into our bodies. As they contract, the lungs then also protect our inner world from harm, creating a loving boundary and expelling anything that may be harmful. This boundary is not only loving, but also flexible, able to change the level of expansion and contraction depending on needs and environmental circumstances. When the lungs are strong, they are able to distinguish positive influences from negative ones and able to say to the negative ones, "No, I do not want this in my body or around me."

Wisdom traditions often relate the lungs to our ability to have a strong sense of self, which includes self-respect and self-value. When we know who we are, we can have good and loving boundaries that enable us to know ourselves as an individual, yet also be open, respectful, and loving with others. We do not "lose" ourselves in someone else or something else, as our identity and self-esteem are secure. We do not eat unhealthy foods, for instance, as we value our physical body.

Balance in the lungs manifests as strong vitality, a powerful voice, and a strong sense of self. We feel and appear strong, as we walk around with an expanded and proud chest and are able to speak with ease and clarity. When out of balance, in contrast, we may appear weak, develop respiratory problems, have a tendency to be sad, have low self-esteem, or be highly judgmental and unable to understand boundaries. To cover up for low self-esteem, we may express false pride and often feel alone and separate from others, unable to feel whole or set in our place in the world. We may be too fanatical about cleanliness or an outright slob, overly disciplined and inflexible or completely unreliable. Most of all, we feel incomplete and become attached to people, places, or things or seek approval from others. We either lose the function of discrepancy or we are too critical. We might *crave* cleanliness and find that being in a messy environment makes us feel like we cannot breathe.

You see, the lungs flourish with health when everything that is unnecessary is eliminated or stored away, and space is created for breathing and reflection. Wisdom traditions describe this as similar to what happens in nature, when fall makes way for winter to come.

> *It is autumn.*
> *The leaves are changing color*
> *and the world is filled with the beauty*
> *of reds, yellows, and oranges.*
> *A gentle breeze fills the air.*
> *I breathe.*
> *Leaves gracefully glide down to the earth.*
> *Winter will soon approach.*
> *Leaves will die, and the trees will be bare.*
> *I hold my breath in this realization.*
> *I then remember.*
> *The leaves will feed the earth.*
> *Spring will bring new beginnings and growth.*
> *I breathe again.*
> *Creation, growth, loss, death, and re-creation.*
> *Thus is the cycle of nature and that of my breath.*
> *I cannot stop the cycle even if I try.*
>
> *I breathe and I am.*
> *I breathe and I am not.*
> *I breathe and find peace*
> *in all that I am*
> *and with all that I have.*

The lungs enjoy beauty, rituals, tradition, and higher virtues and principles—everything that allows for order and space, rather than chaos and destruction. So if you have sensitive or weak lungs, you may find yourself either a clean freak or a slob.

In the Vedic tradition, the lungs occupy the same energy center as the heart, and therefore the two work very closely together. By clearing out negative influences and creating space, the lungs enable the heart to stay open and connected to other people, to one's higher self and purpose, and to the breath of life itself. When the lungs are weakened, the heart is surrounded by negativity and lacks space and confidence to open, leading to a feeling of separateness and disconnection from others, self, and the larger universe.

Bringing Science and Wisdom Traditions Together

Your lungs function by expanding and contracting, taking in oxygen and positivity, if you will, and releasing toxins and negativity. If you think about the movement of expansion and contraction, you can liken expansion to going out in the world and expressing yourself, arms wide open, and exclaiming, "Here I am!" Contraction, on the other hand, represents retreating back into your nest of security and into yourself, putting up a wall between yourself and the world, or going back, if you will, into the womb. Healthy lungs promote your ability to feel centered, confident, and whole as you go out in the world, letting in only whatever helps you thrive and discarding anything that doesn't serve you and your life.

Your lungs are as strong as your sense of self. Have you grown to be confident in yourself, no matter what the situation? Or do you feel more valued because you are driving a new car? Or are popular? Or have a perfect body? Or have a spouse? Is your sense of self-value determined by external factors? Can you be secure and confident without them, let's say, if you lost your job?

If you were brought up to feel valued and encouraged to be the unique person you are with independent likes and thoughts, your sense of self, the ability to feel "whole," would likely be intact. You would be able to mine your weaknesses and harness your strength without taking failure or success personally. You would be able to take in the good, let go of the bad, and allow life's circumstances to bring you to your best place rather than your worst. You would be quite resilient.

Ideally, children grow up in an environment where they are nurtured, loved, and supported to learn, grow, and discover who they are and to feel valued for being unique individuals. They are given structure, yet also freedom to explore. Did you have such an ideal upbringing?

Most likely, in some shape or form, you, like many others, experienced criticism, loss, overprotection, overindulgence, or even abuse. Critical parents, loss, abandonment, or other difficult circumstances may have led you to feel "not enough," so that eventually as an adult you may be overly self-critical, attached to people, places, things, or addictions, or fearful of being alone, of not being loved or safe.

Most of us did not have a perfect childhood and none of us live in a perfect world, so it is likely your sense of self or wholeness can use some polishing. In other words, at some point in your life, you experienced loss, hurt, or lack of support for your beliefs, desires, or choices by someone or by society. According to wisdom traditions, your lungs thus took a hit. You want to keep these ideas in mind as you move farther into learning how to POWER up your lungs, asking yourself such questions as:

How strong is my sense of self?

How confident am I in believing I can go out in the world and express myself?

How do I determine how worthy or valued I am?

Do I tend to be overly critical of myself or others?

Do I tend to withdraw often?

How good am I at saying no to people or things (including food) that do not serve me well?

At sixty-two, Sandra had high blood pressure, high cholesterol, allergies, and her major reason for seeing me, asthma. She reported having had asthma since childhood and that it had worsened over the past year. Sandra denied ever smoking. Her only addiction, she admitted, was overeating comfort food that usually contained a lot of sugar, fat, and artificial additives, which she had turned to recently to cope with stress.

Sandra explained that she had been extremely stressed, because her partner had been very ill earlier in the year, and even though he had recovered, he was still withdrawn and distant. Sandra explained that she had been divorced from her husband for ten years now and in this new relationship for almost two years. Her husband had left her for another woman, and it had taken her years to recover. But now she was very much in love with her new partner, and she was afraid of losing him. First she was scared that she would not survive his being ill, and now she was unsure what was going on because he was so withdrawn.

I asked Sandra to bring her awareness to her chest and tell me what she felt when she thought about losing her partner.

"I feel a big sense of loss. I feel short of breath, a tightness. I want to cry. I feel raw and open. I see myself back in my marriage, and I feel abandoned. I feel unloved and not good enough." Sandra began to cry.

When Sandra was ready, I instructed her to ask her body to show her when she had experienced this feeling before.

She said, "I see myself as a child, forever trying to please my father to ensure his temper would not be set off. It was never enough, and I dared not argue or speak up, because my brother always did and he always got in trouble." Through this exercise, Sandra was able to connect the feeling of being short of breath with her fear of being abandoned, unloved, and her fear of speaking or expressing her truth.

Aside from helping Sandra design a healthy nutrition and exercise program and to see food as fuel rather than comfort, I instructed her on creating new outlets of relief for self-soothing. I suggested she work with a couples therapist who could facilitate better communication with her partner and use healing meditations to help her let go of her feelings of abandonment and, instead, take in feelings of inclusion, love, and appreciation for her full breadth of life.

Today Sandra's relationship has blossomed, and the two are married. She rarely has to use her asthma medications, and she follows a healthy nutrition and exercise plan, on which she lost close to 25 pounds (over a six-month period). At sixty-six, she feels healthier today than she did twenty years ago.

WITNESS the Physiology of Your Lungs

"Witnessing" the lungs is not entirely different from witnessing the heart, but you want to closely observe how the rhythm, quality, and length of the breath change as different emotions or memories arise. You can also observe how the pattern of your breath influences your thoughts, emotions, and memories.

For example, I tend to get exercise-induced asthma. On occasion, if I have been exposed to a virus, I might experience more asthma during exercise, though not when I am inactive. I can tell, however, that my lungs are weaker, because I tend to be more emotional or sad without much good reason. In addition, when I am sad or upset, I tend to be more susceptible to colds or to a flare-up of asthma during exercise.

Now try to notice how your breath might change in response to positive or negative imagery or thoughts. Pay attention to the pace or rhythm of your breathing, the length of the breath, especially the out-flow, and whether you feel a tightness or a sense of ease.

AWARENESS EXERCISE

Close your eyes, and begin with the practice of emptying the mind.

If you can, try breathing only through your nose at first. Notice the air as it moves in and out. Notice the rhythm and quality of your breath.

Then bring your awareness to your chest, and notice what you feel there. Do you notice any emotion in particular?

Breathe through your mouth now and notice what you feel as the air moves in and out. Pay attention to the rhythm or even the temperature of the air.

Bring your awareness back to your chest, and notice what you feel and if any particular emotions are present.

Shift your focus to your abdomen, and allow the abdomen to inflate like a balloon as you inhale and deflate as you exhale. Notice the rhythm and quality of your breath.

Come back to your chest and notice what you feel and if you feel any particular emotions.

Does your chest feel open, closed, relaxed, tight, heavy, or light? Where? Notice.

What happens with your breath when you experience or think about the following (take your time with each one):

The slow rhythm of the ocean waves, in and out

A fast-paced walk downtown to get to a meeting

Walking on a path in nature and admiring its beauty

Being stuck in traffic and late to work

A situation that has left you sad or heartbroken

A situation that has left you feeling proud and thankful

A feeling of being devastated and unlucky

A feeling of being the luckiest person in the world

Did you notice how your breath changed with different images or thoughts? Did you observe feeling differently when the focus of your breathing changed?

The lungs are strongly connected to your emotions and the regulation of your stress response, just like the heart. Whether you suffer from lung problems or not, it is unlikely that you have led an injury-free life, as we all breathe the same air, and most of us—at least I still do—have work to do on feeling whole and complete within ourselves. So I invite you now to examine further what you may have felt or experienced just now in this witnessing exercise.

EXAMINE Your Deeper Emotions and Beliefs

Perhaps you can examine your lungs for yourself by seeing how each of these statements makes you feel and respond. Note which of the following statements elicit the strongest emotional response, whether it is avoidance or resonance. As you do so, keep in mind the functions of the lungs: contraction and expansion, contracting to expel the negativity, then expanding to take in what will restore, renew, and protect. Sometimes there is an imbalance on the expansion, or letting in, side;

people let too much in and seek value externally. An imbalance on the contraction, or letting go, side causes people to be closed and to retreat from the world. Imbalances on both sides represent weaker lung function and result in rigidity, the need to control, and being judgmental. The virtues of openness, flexibility, ease in expressing oneself, and appreciation represent strong lung functions.

Imbalance in Expansion:

I often find myself in situations where I feel helpless and wish I could be rescued.

I am often very emotional or needy and seek attention or advice, as I do not trust my own feelings or know what to do.

I am often surrounded by chaos.

I often care excessively about what others think.

I am adamant about saying that I don't care about what others think.

I often need approval from others.

Imbalance in Contraction:

I often feel like an imposter.

I am often hypersensitive to the thoughts or statements of others.

I am sometimes seen as an "ice princess" or "stuffed shirt."

I rarely ask for help and tend to withdraw.

I rarely speak up, even if I have something to say.

I worry I will be criticized often.

Imbalance in Expansion and Contraction:

I tend to need my surroundings to be in perfect order and clean, or else I feel anxious.

I am a stickler for routine.

I can be self-righteous and judgmental when others act in a way that upsets me.

I often need to be in control.

I tend to be possessive when it comes to people or my material things.

Once you have read these statements, choose two or three that elicit the strongest response and do the following exercise.

GOING DEEPER EXERCISE

Begin with the practice of emptying the mind.

Bring your awareness to your chest and your breath. Observe what you feel. What happens to your breath—is it long, short, constricted, fluid, and so on?

What sort of emotion are you experiencing, if any at all?

As you observe, ask yourself when you became this way, and why.

Ask yourself where you learned that you were not valued enough that you had to _____ (fill in)?

Ask yourself why you need to be this way.

Notice what comes up for you—thoughts, images, emotions, memories, and so on—and then write them down.

RELEASE, RELIEVE, and RESTORE

There are many ways to keep your lungs healthy and strong, and you have already begun to do so by learning more about the lungs and starting the process of releasing whatever negativity you are holding on to. As you go farther in this process, remember that for the lungs to be healthy, you want to create a clean, loving, and open environment for them inside and out. You also want to work on knowing your own inner strength and value, knowing when to be out in the world and when to rest and renew.

If you do have an existing lung condition or severe or persistent symptoms, please follow up with your health-care provider to ensure that while your breathing is unstable, you are on appropriate medications, such as a steroid or an albuterol inhaler, antibiotics, or even oxygen if necessary. Your goal is to either be able to get off medications or need to use them only minimally.

The good news is that "the lungs are very durable if they're not attacked from the outside," according to Norman H. Edelman, M.D., chief medical officer of the American Lung Association.[9] So put a stop to the attack now.

Creating a Clean and Loving Environment

As you breathe in and out during the following exercise, be aware that your lungs are deeply intertwined with your emotions, beliefs, and thoughts as well as your heart. Negative thoughts, emotions, and beliefs connect with hurts in your heart, causing your lungs to work hard to get rid of the toxins, just as they get rid of carbon dioxide and take in oxygen. Your lungs want you to take in the good and expel the bad.

HEALING MEDITATION

Bring your awareness to your breath and your chest.

Notice how your chest feels as you breathe in and out. Is it open or closed, relaxed or tight, heavy or light?

What is the quality of your breath? Is it fluid, smooth, constricted, short, fast, slow, long?

There is no right or wrong, you are simply observing what you feel.

So let go now. Exhale, and release all that doesn't serve you into the wind.

Let go of negative beliefs, thoughts, or emotions that make you feel "less than."

Let go of grief, loss, heaviness, or longing.

Let go and make space.

Breathe in and breathe in space. Breathe in oxygen. Breathe in the breath of life.

Breathe in the wisdom of the universe.

Breathe in the ebb and flow of nature.

Breathe in your own uniqueness.

Breathe so that your heart opens to the breath of life.

Breathe in your wholeness.

Breathe in and out, the ebb and flow of life.

In and out.

TEARS: Cry if you need to. According to science, crying can make people feel better and reduce stress.[10] In traditional Chinese medicine, the lungs are associated with the feelings of loss and grief and therefore tears represent a form of cleansing and release. Use your tears as an opportunity to find meaning, as you let go of feelings of loss and make room for growth and connection. You may choose to journal within or on paper; also do the witnessing and examining exercises. Give yourself the space to grieve and to cry. Often the minute you love yourself enough to give yourself permission to cry, the crying stops as soon as it starts.

A CLEAN ENVIRONMENT: Your lungs function better with less clutter and pollution around. You may actually find that you breathe easier when you organize your immediate environments like your home or your office. So clean out your closets, cupboards, desks, or finances. You can hire someone to help you if necessary.

You may also benefit from having an air purifier in the places you spend more time, like your bedroom, especially if you have asthma or other lung conditions. If possible, aim to avoid places where the air is too cold or hot or polluted with irritants like smoke, dust, chemical fumes (even those used at home like paints and solvents), or asbestos. If you have a product that has a label warning that it may cause skin or eye irritation, try to avoid using it, but if you have to, wear a mask and eye protection. You may also want to find out if your home or workplace has radon to avoid exposure to that as well; go to www.epa.gov/radon to find out how to deal with radon.

Staying Strong with Regular Exercise

Exercise in itself may not contribute directly to the function of the lungs, but when you are more fit, your lungs are more efficient at getting the oxygen in and carbon dioxide out. Your immune system stays stronger, which helps defend you against lung infections. Exercise also helps you increase your lung capacity. You can do aerobics, cycle, power walk, jog, or mix in sprints with walking to give your lungs a good workout. Swimming, in particular, can really help you increase your lung capacity, as research shows that lung capacity is improved when exercises are performed in the water.[11]

Lung Food

A recent study at Barts and the London School of Medicine showed that those individuals who favored fresh fruit and vegetables, oily fish, and whole-grain products had far better lung function than those who chose a diet high in fat, sugar, and processed food.[12] Other studies are finding that people who eat more cruciferous vegetables like broccoli, cauliflower, cabbage, bok choy, kale, and mustard greens have a decreased risk of getting lung cancer compared to those who eat fewer of these vegetables.[13]

Interestingly, traditional Chinese medicine recommends eating more foods like asparagus, broccoli, celery, mustard greens, onions, radishes, rice, almonds, apricots, pears, and bananas (to name a few) and avoiding dairy and sugar to help strengthen lung function. Mustard greens, onions, radishes, and pears, for instance, help clear and eliminate phlegm, while mustard greens also aid in improving energy circulation. Dairy and sugar (including sweeteners) increase mucus or phlegm production. In other wisdom traditions, a combination of chopped onions and honey does the trick in clearing congestion and phlegm, while vegetables improve energy flow.

When you are trying to figure out which foods to eat and which to avoid, think about foods that are nurturing and warming, but not heavy. Dairy, sugar, white-flour products, and processed foods are "heavy" and highly inflammatory. Eating such foods will cause stress on your system and weigh down your lungs. As a general rule then, you want to do the following:

- Eat plenty of vegetables, especially green ones for all the reasons you have learned so far—fiber, antioxidants, vitamins, and minerals. Go green, go lungs!

- Eat oily fish, which will provide you with vitamin D and omega-3 fatty acids. In fact, low vitamin-D levels have been associated with worsening lung function and chronic lung disease, so it behooves you to have these levels checked and make sure you are getting adequate amounts of vitamin D in general.[14]

- Eat orange fruits and vegetables, like carrots and oranges, which provide vitamins A, C, and B6 and a variety of antioxidants. Scientific studies show that carrots and other foods rich in antioxidants like vitamin C can help people avoid lung deterioration and prevent lung infections like pneumonia.[15]

- Eat onions, which are rich in sulfur compounds that are highly antibacterial. When my aunt told me to drink hot water with onions and honey for my cold, I thought, "Yuck!" But it worked. Onions also have expectorant properties, which help the body get rid of phlegm. In addition to vitamins C and B6 and other nutrients, onions also have quercetin, a natural antioxidant that can aid in reducing the inflammation that may accompany allergies and asthma. Research is also finding that quercetin may be helpful in preventing lung cancer.[16]

- Eat foods that help restore your body's natural flora, or friendly bacteria and also help you reduce inflammation and phlegm: for example, fermented foods, as you learned in the immune system chapter.

Social Support and Counseling

As is true for your general health, social support enables you to feel stronger, take better care of yourself, and feel less alone. Lungs represent the need to feel safe in order to express yourself, so what better way to achieve this than by having people to talk to, feel safe around, and laugh with. As the lungs are often negatively affected by loss or grief, I find working with a therapist, counselor, or minister or being in a support group can facilitate the healing process.

Join a support group, book club, or interest group. Ask a friend to help you make sure you feel safe to express yourself. Work with a therapist if necessary, especially if you are trying to work through loss.

Connecting with Your Sense of Self, Nurturance, and Value

APPRECIATION AND EXPRESSION: Just as deciduous trees must lose their leaves, you cannot hold on to the past or your possessions, but you can hold on to your sense of self and your ability to appreciate, honor, and connect to higher truths and purposes. One way of doing so is by practicing mindfulness, or staying present and connected, in a state of appreciation, as much as possible. I particularly find taking a mindful walk in nature helpful in achieving the goal of feeling more connected not only to the big picture of life, but to the appreciation of my role in it.

You can make walking in nature part of your daily routine, connecting with the beauty and perfection of all things, so that ultimately you can connect with your own beauty and perfection. Joining with nature also allows you to appreciate the ebb and flow of life and, ultimately, to learn how to let go and allow in, as nature does. After all, nature not only lets a flower bloom, but also lets a forest burn as a way of making room for new growth.

I remember a personal experience of turning to nature when I lost a dear friend on the same day that a patient awoke after having a heart transplant. My walk enabled me to open to appreciation as well as make space to express my grief. Finding ways to express yourself, in general, can help you move into appreciation and also find your "self" or your voice. You can take voice lessons, classes in public speaking, creative writing, dance, or painting, for example.

REST BREAKS AND SLEEP: As you have learned already, sleep and rest are essential for the health of your mind and body, the strength of your immune system, and your ability to recuperate and manage stress. Many individuals with lung problems may have difficulty sleeping, especially if the symptoms are active at night, like with asthma. Some individuals may also have sleep apnea, a condition in which one stops breathing momentarily and the oxygen supply is cut off. If you have a sleeping partner, you may want to ask if you snore very loudly and if there are intermittent pauses in your breathing, especially if you are awakening feeling tired, have frequent headaches, cannot stay awake during the day, cannot lose weight, or have developed high blood pressure. If you have any of these symptoms, do visit your doctor for an evaluation. In the meantime, take naps when you can and practice your breath work.

BREATH PRACTICE: You can also do gentle exercises like yoga and tai chi, which focus on breathing practices. You can do breath work with or without movement. You can practice one of the following:

> Imagine there is a balloon in your abdomen that is expanding as you inhale and deflating as you exhale.

Breathe in slowly through your nose and even more slowly out through your mouth, through lips that are almost closed, so it takes longer for the air to leave. This is teaching your lungs to be able to hold on to air longer and stretching out the sacs.

Breathe in for a count of four, then hold your breath for a count of four, and then exhale for a count of six or for as long as you can in order to empty your lungs.

CHAPTER SEVEN

The Gastrointestinal System

You Eat and You Are

I was always happy when he was around. My
heart did not stay still in its place even. Nowadays
my stomach replaced my heart. I was filling my
stomach as long as my heart stayed empty. Just
because of filling somewhere inside of me.

—ARZUM UZUN, *NERDESIN ASKIM*

The stomach and digestive system have been used throughout time and across cultures to depict the emotional, mental,
or physical state of the body and mind. Saying a person has
"a strong stomach" implies one who can withstand watching or con-
fronting hardship, while "the pit of the stomach" is described as the
location of anxiety; "trusting your gut" means trusting your instincts.
Science now confirms that you actually do "feel" from your gut and
has deemed its neural circuitry a "second brain," one that produces

neurotransmitters like serotonin and often works independently of the actual brain.

The gastrointestinal tract is about thirty feet in length and performs a whole host of functions that enable you to survive and thrive. These functions include the ability to digest, to break down and absorb nutrients, and to eliminate waste and other substances that do not serve your well-being. If your digestive system is weak, you cannot digest or utilize nutrients to the maximum benefit. This is akin to being sleep deprived and sitting in an interesting lecture. It doesn't matter how wonderful the lecturer is, you will not listen attentively, fully absorb the lesson, or be able to integrate the lesson into your life. When you support your digestive system, you reinforce your own vital energy and your ability to fully access what you need to have a vibrant life.

Modern Western dietary habits negatively affect the digestive system in a variety of ways. Think about it. Most food has to be broken down to be utilized by the microscopic cells of your body. It must be divided into smaller molecules, so that it can be absorbed into the bloodstream and delivered to the internal organs and brain for energy. Foods that are processed, unnatural, or filled with chemicals require a lot more work to break down. In addition, gulping down food and swallowing whole rather than chewing, as we tend to do when we are on the run, create a bigger burden on your pancreas because it has to provide enzymes to break down whole food all at once, rather than food that has been partially broken down and mixed with saliva in your mouth. Given our modern Western eating habits, can you imagine then how hard the system has to work to make half of what Americans eat nourishing? What we eat, how we eat it, and why we eat it really warrant closer examination—and change.

For starters, we have to remember that food is meant to nourish and fuel, not to satisfy or deal with emotions. Every part of the gastrointestinal system has a purpose and function—whether it is to ingest, discriminate and protect, absorb and integrate, or eliminate—to help us be alive in a vibrant way. When you really understand and strengthen these functions, not only will your gastrointestinal system become more resilient, but so will you.

This chapter will guide you as you:

- Press the PAUSE button and become acquainted with the anatomy and functions of the gastrointestinal system.

- OPTIMIZE your awareness of the digestive system by learning about what can go wrong, the signs and symptoms to watch out for that tell you to get medical help, and the bigger picture the gastrointestinal tract represents when viewed by wisdom traditions.

- Discover how your digestive system might be speaking to you as you WITNESS your physiology through guided exercises.

- EXAMINE underlying emotions or beliefs that may be weakening your ability to fully digest, absorb, discriminate, or eliminate not only food and waste products, but also ideas, beliefs, or experiences.

- Develop the tools that will help you RELEASE negative habits and beliefs that do not nurture you, RELIEVE your body of stress and toxins, and RESTORE your gastrointestinal system back to its powerful and resilient state.

PAUSE and OPTIMIZE Your Awareness of Your Digestive System

Anatomy and Functions

Digestion actually starts with your nose, as your sense of smell allows you to determine what you want to eat. Once you put the food into your mouth and chew, saliva containing special enzymes like amylase is secreted by three pairs of salivary glands to help break down the food.

As you chew, the food becomes mush, which is called a bolus. The tongue moves the bolus up and backward so that it reaches the back of the throat. When you swallow, muscles move the bolus down and to the back of the esophagus. The muscles of the esophagus then move the food down to the stomach. So that food can enter the stomach without allowing a backward flow of acid, at the end of the esophagus is a ring-like muscle, called the lower esophageal sphincter, that constricts and effectively separates the esophagus from the stomach, once the food is in the stomach.

Once in there, the stomach muscles work to move the bolus around so that it can mix with and be dissolved by hydrochloric acid and gastric juices filled with powerful enzymes such as pepsin. Once the task is complete, the stomach empties its contents in the form of liquid or paste into the small intestine.

About twenty feet long, the small intestine is made up of three sections: duodenum, jejunum, and ileum. As the muscles of the duodenum contract, the bolus mixes with enzymes released from the pancreas and bile from the liver. The enzymes of the pancreas help break down carbohydrates, proteins, and fat, while bile acids produced in the liver, which are stored in and then secreted from the gallbladder, serve to break down fat. Since fat is too large of a molecule for the pancreatic enzymes to break down on their own, bile acids emulsify the fat, acting like a detergent that causes fat globules to break down into smaller droplets or particles. Pancreatic lipase can then break these droplets down even further.

Absorption of nutrients begins in the small intestine, mostly in the jejunum and ileum. Nutrients like calcium, magnesium, iron, vitamin A, vitamin D, and glucose are absorbed in the duodenum. Fat, sucrose, lactose (from milk), vitamin B6, thiamine, vitamin B2 and vitamin C, folic acid, and B12 are absorbed in the ileum.

Leftover by-products—whatever is not absorbed in the small intestine—are delivered to the colon, or large intestine, which is about five to six feet in length. The by-products move from the cecum to the right, or ascending (upward), colon; to the transverse (horizontal) colon; down the left, or descending (downward), colon; to the S-shaped sigmoid colon; and to the rectum. Water, potassium, sodium, and fatty acids from fiber are absorbed along the way until the liquid bolus becomes formed stool, a combination of undigested food parts, old mucosal cells, and bacteria, which is ultimately stored in the rectum, where it accumulates until it is pushed out (also known as a bowel movement).

Gas or stool in the rectum sends messages to the brain to stimulate the muscles of the rectum to contract, while relaxing the muscles of the anal sphincter, so that contents can be released and passed through the anus to create the bowel movement. You actually have two anal sphincters, an internal sphincter, which works without your conscious thought (like keeping the stool in while you are sleeping), and an external sphincter, which you can control voluntarily.

A complex feedback loop of hormone signals and enzymes enables you to digest, absorb, and eliminate food. Protein in your stomach, for example, stimulates pepsin to be released as well as histamine. As the pepsin starts breaking down the protein, gastrin signals nearby cells to release acid, the muscles of the stomach to contract, and the muscles of the pyloric sphincter to relax (located between the stomach and the small intestine). As the protein is broken down into smaller amino acids, more hormones, digestive enzymes, and acid are released. The higher the acid in the stomach, the more gastrin is released. Once the acid level drops, and this is usually because the contents have now moved on to the intestine, gastrin levels fall.

It is important that the high acid level of the stomach contents be neutralized as they enter the duodenum. To make this happen, the hormone secretin is secreted by the cells of the duodenum to signal the pancreas to send out its digestive juices filled with bicarbonate. Secretin also stimulates the release of bile from the liver and signals the stomach secretions and contractions to stop.

Meanwhile, other hormones are released in the small intestine, some to signal the gallbladder to empty and others to cause the sphincter lying between the liver-pancreas and duodenum to relax and open, the release of insulin from the pancreas, and feeding to be either resumed or stopped. The functions and activities of these hormones are highly influenced by sight, smell, taste, thoughts, stress, emotional states, and adaptive behavior patterns. For example, anxiety, fear, or illness can trigger activity in the sympathetic nervous system, or the release of adrenalin, which suppresses contraction and secretion of gastric juices, induces relaxation instead, and lessens blood flow to the gut, thus shutting digestion down. Normally, an individual's appetite would be suppressed too. However, let's say that you have developed the habit of eating more food to help you handle stress. In this case the normal feedback loop that tells your brain to stop eating and shut down your appetite is turned off. Instead, the signal essentially says, "Eat, you will feel better," even though your nervous system is also signaling your digestive system to shut down. The result is that you eat more food and end up getting an upset stomach.

In other words, your gut is closely linked to your stress response and the associated coping habits. Changes in mood affect your food intake, and your food intake, in turn, influences your mood. Have you experienced gastrointestinal upset when stressed? How about that nervousness in the "pit" of your stomach?

Many years ago when I was still working in the hospital, I used to experience terrible stomach pains every time I had to have interactions with a senior physician who seemed not to share my ideas about how to treat patients more holistically. My first inclination was to develop a strong dislike toward this doctor, but that did not work for me either, because I also respected him and the knowledge he could impart to me. Every time I got mad, my stomach hurt more and my desire to eat baked goods increased. So instead of eating yet another chocolate chip muffin, I reflected on the discomfort in my stomach. I asked myself why was I experiencing pain there. My gut literally told me that my sense of self-worth was being challenged—not by the senior physician, but by me. I was the one doubting my ideas and beliefs. This physician was simply challenging me on my own assertions. As I worked on believing in myself, the symptoms ceased, as did my cravings for muffins.

Of course, not everyone who experiences stomach pain will have the same issues, nor is it guaranteed that, once you address the emotional issues that are being triggered, the symptoms will go away. Your gastrointestinal system is actually very resilient, but because it is constantly being barraged by what you ingest, it is at high risk for damage, both structurally and functionally.

What Can Go Wrong

HIGH ACID IN THE WRONG PLACES: Obstructive tumors, poor dentition, poor food choices, or simply the aging process can negatively affect the gastrointestinal system. As you age, for example, the acidity in the stomach starts to drop. Low acid levels hinder proper digestion and trigger gastrin levels to rise. This leads to more stomach muscle contraction as well as relaxation of the esophageal sphincter, resulting in a reflux of gastric juices into the esophagus, causing a high acid level in a place where it should be low. Stress and poor food choices, such as alcohol, highly processed foods, and foods high in sugar and chemical additives, can upset the balance of the gastrin feedback loop, resulting in heartburn, indigestion, reflux disease, or inflammation and destruction of the stomach (gastritis) or esophageal lining (esophagitis).

LOW ACID WHERE IT IS SUPPOSED TO BE HIGH: If gastrin levels are low, the stomach has difficulty breaking down B12 for absorption in the ileum. Low B12 levels can lead to a whole host of problems, including fatigue, poor cognitive functioning, depression, or other neurological symptoms.

GLITCHES IN THE HORMONE FEEDBACK LOOP: With stress, poor food choices, poor coping habits, medications, or preexisting medical conditions, the hormonal feedback loop can get disrupted. Take sleep deprivation, for example. Studies show that lack of sleep (less than six hours a night) is related to increase in appetite and hunger for high-fat and high-carbohydrate foods.[1] Normally, with adequate sleep, the hormone ghrelin is released to stimulate hunger when you are truly in need of food, and leptin is released when you are full or satiated, to suppress your hunger. With loss of sleep this signaling system is disrupted, and leptin levels fall and ghrelin levels rise. Have you ever found yourself sleep deprived and craving sweet or fatty food? This is why, and it is just one example of hormonal mayhem. Lack of sleep also triggers more activation of the stress response and higher adrenalin and cortisol levels, which then affect all systems of the body. Acid levels may fall or rise, esophageal contractions may be stimulated, or the contractions of the intestinal muscles may be inhibited. You might then experience irritable bowel syndrome or heartburn when the intestinal lining takes a beating.

Facts for You to Digest

- More than 34 million Americans are afflicted with diseases of the digestive system; 20 million with chronic diseases.

- As a group, the digestive diseases account for 8–9 percent of total U.S. mortality, with 60 percent of digestive-disease mortality due to malignant neoplasms and 40 percent to nonmalignant causes, chief of which is cirrhosis of the liver.

- Digestive diseases are the second leading cause of disability due to illness in the United States. Digestive diseases are the leading cause of time lost from work for male employees, and account for 15 percent of all absences from work among workers ages seventeen to sixty-four.

- The total economic cost associated with digestive diseases has been estimated at more than $50 billion annually.[2]

DAMAGE TO THE LINING: Damage to the intestinal lining, which can occur because of poor food choices, high- or low-acid levels, or chronic activation of the stress response, can result in a whole host of problems that interrupt the hormonal feedback loop, digestion, absorption, and the bowel movement itself. Such damage can also result in destruction of the natural bacteria that live in the gastrointestinal tract. These friendly bacteria help you digest and absorb nutrients, maintain a good pH, and fight infection. Without them, disease-forming bacteria can take over, and a variety of complications can arise, such as bloating, ulcers, irregularity, achiness, and fatigue.

The point is that when or if you experience gastrointestinal issues, there are usually multiple factors involved. It is a "system" after all, and when the system fails or is injured, you can experience a myriad of problems from dental caries to heartburn, ulcers, and gallstones; infection or inflammation of the gallbladder, liver, pancreas, or colon; collapse or out-pouching of the gut lining (as in hemorrhoids); or cancer.

Usually, most gastrointestinal problems are intermittent, less severe, and easily treated or prevented, as you will soon discover. Having said that, visit with your health-care provider when you do have symptoms, as the likelihood is that there is a treatable solution, and definitely seek medical attention immediately if you have any of these red flags.

Red Flags That Tell You to Get Help

Though most common GI issues are usually intermittent and symptoms typically resolve when treated, some symptoms and signs indicate red flags, or serious warnings to seek medical attention immediately.

- Unusual, persistent, or excruciating abdominal pain

- Bloody or black-tarry stools

- Bloody vomit

- Heartburn that is severe or getting worse and is not relieved with medication

- Pain that is interfering with daily activities

- Difficulty swallowing

- Persistent hoarseness or sore throat

- Persistent diarrhea

- New and persistent constipation

- Periods of choking

- Unexplained weight loss

At forty-five years old, Jessie had never been married and had never really had a serious relationship. For the most part, she said, she was perfectly happy, as she had many friends, took a lot of adventurous trips throughout the world, and enjoyed her job. She came to me not to find a boyfriend, but because even though she was "happy," she had problems with anxiety and sleep disturbance and, more irritatingly, problems with her stomach that were interfering with her life of adventure. She complained that her stomach was always "upset," which manifested in cramping and diarrhea, which then affected her energy level. She denied eating junk food and said she ate a "healthy diet," which included cereal with skim milk and fruit in the morning, cereal for her snack, and a variety of proteins and vegetables, including cheese and yogurt for the rest of her meals.

As part of her first homework assignment, I asked Jessie to keep a food and symptom journal addressing such questions as: How do you feel the next day after eating dairy? Do you experience any stiffness of your joints, and if so, when and what have you eaten that day or the day before? On the days that you do not eat cereal, how do you feel? What happens to your stomach when you feel anxious? How does this affect your food choices? When you think about being in a relationship, do you feel anxious or calm and what happens to your stomach?

When Jessie returned with her journal, she had become aware of some conclusions. Her stomach usually felt lousy after eating dairy. Her joints always ached and were stiff in the morning, and she felt less tired on days she did not consume cereal. Her anxiety always seemed to be tied in with her stomach upset, and just thinking about being in a relationship caused her stomach to be bound up.

Now that Jessie was more in tune with the effects food had on her body and the affects her emotions had on her food choices and symptoms, I asked Jessie to close her eyes, think about being in a relationship, and tell me what she was feeling in her stomach in that very moment. I then guided her through an awareness exercise to see what her stomach could tell us:

> DR. EVA: Jessie, can you tell me what you are feeling right now in your stomach?
>
> JESSIE: I am feeling tension, like my stomach cannot relax.
>
> DR. EVA: If you were to flash a light on the area of tension, what would it appear like?
>
> JESSIE: It looks like a bound-up ball of energy.
>
> DR. EVA: If you were to get close and notice what sort of emotion is being released from this ball of energy, can you tell me what it is?
>
> JESSIE: I am sensing fear, sadness, and disappointment.

DR. EVA: Why? Can you ask the ball of energy why it is there? Is it there to protect you from something? When did you first create it?

JESSIE: It is there to protect. I first created it in middle school. I felt unattractive. Boys did not like me. I was very alone. I spent time finding other things to do. I made up adventures.

DR. EVA: Was that a bad thing to do?

JESSIE: I should have tried to fit in. I was different.

DR. EVA: As an adult, Jessie, and looking back now, is it really bad to be different and adventurous? Were you really unwanted or unattractive? How do you perceive being adventurous now?

JESSIE: No, it is not bad. It is a good trait. I like that trait.

DR. EVA: So you can tell little Jessie that and let her know she is not bad or unworthy and that she can use her trait as an asset, not as an escape. She can share this asset with other people openly, and they will love her back. Do your friends not love you now, Jessie?

JESSIE: They do.

DR. EVA: How does little Jessie feel now?

JESSIE: Happy.

DR. EVA: What are you feeling in your stomach at the thought of being in a relationship?

JESSIE: Nothing. It feels relaxed. I feel open.

For the next few months, Jessie continued to work through distorted beliefs related to her self-esteem and fear of rejection. At the same time, she worked on rebuilding her digestive system, improving her diet, and reinstating the natural bacteria that needed to line her gut. Jessie removed all gluten and dairy from her diet and ate mostly grass-fed proteins, fish, vegetables, and some fruits. She started on fish-oil and vitamin-D supplements as well as probiotics to help with digestion, absorption, and mood.

Perhaps you can see from Jessie's story that there is a lot more to the gastrointestinal system than simply eating food and having bowel movements.

What Wisdom Traditions Say About Digestion

According to wisdom traditions, a strong body and a healthy digestive system represent your ability to be in harmony and agreeability with the earth, your surroundings, others, and yourself. In the five-element system of traditional Chinese medicine, your spleen is the organ mainly responsible for digestion and nourishment and is associated with the element of earth, or Mother Earth, if you will. To best understand this concept, think about what Mother Earth does. She is responsible for ingesting, digesting, and assimilating the earth's materials so they can be used to support new life, like taking the dead leaves that fall from the trees to fertilize the soil for new growth.

Your spleen, according to traditional Chinese medicine (not Western medicine), provides nourishment and warmth to your body. It regulates your metabolism and supports the integrity of the body, while providing you with energy. Your spleen is also involved in the digestion of your ideas and the extraction of new information from your experiences. It influences your ability to reflect, think creatively, innovate, concentrate, and assimilate stressful experiences into opportunities for self-growth. According to this wisdom tradition, when your gas-trointestinal system is not in balance, you might experience digestive problems, but you may also incur other symptoms such as worry, feel-ings of being overwhelmed, poor concentration, rigid thinking, lack of creativity, or a poor sense of self or self-worth.

The Vedic tradition has a similar approach. The third, or solar plexus, chakra (recall that chakras are energy centers responsible for transforming spiritual energy into physical energy) is associated with digestion and the corresponding organs. This chakra is located be-tween the rib cage and navel and governs the upper abdomen, stom-ach, spleen, intestine, liver, pancreas, and gallbladder. It is believed that this energy center governs creative and intuitive abilities as well as the rational side of the mind, assimilation of thoughts, the ego, and expe-riences that help you define yourself. A healthy third chakra represents a healthy digestive system, whereby you know who you are, what is nourishing for you and what is not, and are able to absorb and assimi-late life's experiences in a healthy way, without losing yourself or being destroyed; you are able to let go and be rid of whatever it is that does not serve, help, or better you.

Can you see the correlation now between Jessie's story or my story and the circumstances or emotions that added to the symptoms? In my case, feeling threatened for my beliefs and not really believing in my-self led to stomach distress, while acceptance allowed me to feel better. When the functions of the digestive system—ingestion, discrimina-tion and protection, absorption and integration, and elimination—are healthy, they manifest as a healthy sense of self, the ability to digest and assimilate information and life's lessons, and being able to let go of whatever doesn't serve you. In turn, when these character traits, atti-tudes, or behaviors are strong, your digestive system benefits.

What the Metaphor of Digestion Means for You

You can use the metaphor of digestion and the gastrointestinal system's functions as guides for self-examination and investigation of your needs and how you perceive yourself and your life. When you think about, for example, *ingestion*, you can reflect on how you take in and break down information, ideas, or experiences; *discrimination* and *protection*—how you evaluate what you take in and are able to discriminate between beneficial and harmful elements; *absorption* and *integration*—how you assimilate and integrate fuel made up of ideas and experiences into the rest of the body and your life; and *elimination*—how you remove waste and whatever does not serve you or your body, including thoughts and beliefs.

When these functions are in balance, the following happens:

You know who you are and you do not need to be defined or feel validated by others or external circumstances. You are able to *choose* only what you want and what is nourishing. *Location of benefit:* Entire digestive tract.

You know how to discern between healthy and unhealthy information, people, or thoughts, so that you can sift through your experiences, decisively say no to what hurts you, and take in only what nourishes you. *Location of benefit:* Entire digestive tract, with a focus on the stomach, small intestine, pancreas, liver, and gallbladder, as further breakdown and discernment is involved. Wisdom traditions, in fact, see the gallbladder as representing your *will* and ability to cut to the chase, with surety and gusto.

You are able to take in nourishment and assimilate and integrate it with your whole self, maintaining a strong sense of self-worth and self-esteem. If weak, you are unsure about yourself and you may use outside circumstances to bring comfort to feelings of inadequacy. You invariably then feel worse and the cycle persists. *Location of benefit:* Entire digestive tract, especially the colon and the anus.

You are able to "let go" of whatever thoughts, ideas, or beliefs you might have ingested that do not belong in your body. You are able to stay "clean" in mind and body, not ruminating or holding on to toxins that come from beliefs or words that hurt rather than nourish you. Wisdom traditions connect this function with being strong in your own identity. *Location of benefit:* Entire digestive tract, especially small intestine, where absorption happens, as well as the colon.

Ready to witness the gastrointestinal system for yourself?

WITNESS the Physiology of Your Digestive System

AWARENESS EXERCISE

Breathe in on a count of three. Breathe out on the count of five. Empty the thoughts from your mind (four cycles).

Shift your awareness to your mouth. Notice what you feel. Allow all your senses to be engaged.

Notice how the saliva already starts building up and what that feels like.

Swallow the saliva. Notice the process of swallowing. Be aware of how the saliva moves down your throat, then down the esophagus, then into the stomach.

Notice any sensations you experience along the way. Always breathe in for three, out for five.

Notice what you feel in your stomach. When you breathe, is your stomach feeling tense or relaxed?

Imagine the saliva moving through all the intestines down to your colon, where it is absorbed. Notice what and how you feel as you become aware of the rectum and anus as you breathe in and out.

Breathe in for three, breathe out for five. Notice sensations, emotions, images, or thoughts that may arise with these statements. Make a mental note also where the sensations arise.

I am being recognized for a job well done.

People are talking badly about me behind my back.

I feel stuck and am unable to come up with any new ideas.

I feel alive with creativity and possibilities.

I am fearful of being rejected.

I am warmed at the loving reception my friends had for me.

I am unworthy.

EXAMINE Your Deeper Emotions and Beliefs

I invite you to examine the following statements or questions and notice which one elicits the strongest response in your stomach or any area of your digestive tract. Also, if you tend to have any of the problems mentioned earlier in this chapter, you can focus on that particular symptom or functional problem instead. Perhaps you have a tendency to get constipated or have heartburn; pay attention to that symptom or part of your body. Or you know you have issues with low self-esteem. When you focus on your low self-esteem or situations that cause you to feel unworthy, notice where this might show up as sensations in your abdomen like contraction, tension, or restriction. For instance, you may want to examine the "knot" in your stomach or a feeling of heaviness, of being "blocked," as one can get with constipation.

I tend to please people sometimes at my own expense.

I make sure I take care of myself first and tend to others later. Why shouldn't I?

I often feel that I am being taken for granted.

I often feel that I am not important enough or feel inadequate.

I find myself in situations where I am not valued. Why can't they see me and my worth?

I crave attention and comfort when I am upset and often use food to comfort.

I often find myself saying, "I don't deserve this!"

I have often felt wronged, that something has been taken away from me, and I fight back in response.

I have a hard time making decisions and am not sure what is best for me.

I get angry or upset when I am criticized.

I have a hard time letting go when someone upsets me or criticizes me.

I tend to ruminate and overthink things.

I am grieving loss and cannot seem to let go.

If I let people in close, they always disappoint me.

If I let people in close, they may reject me.

GOING DEEPER EXERCISE

Close your eyes, breathe deeply, and take your time with each statement. See how you or your body reacts, specifically along the digestive tract. Where does the tension or negative sensation appear most?

Feel, look at (with an imaginary flashlight), examine the emitted emotion, ask "Why are you there?" or "When did I first create you?" and allow your imagination or thoughts to carry you to another place and time.

Allow the movie reel to play out and see where it takes you, looking for the time your needs first were not met, that is, your needs to be fueled and nourished, loved, and valued for being you.

When you are ready, write down your experience and how it makes you feel today. Write without holding back and see where the process takes you.

RELEASE, RELIEVE, and RESTORE

The foundation you have been creating can now be used to heal and strengthen not only your digestive system, but your own beliefs, attitudes, and ways of being in life. The aim now is to focus on incorporating tools and activities that enable you to reinforce your ability to ingest nourishment, discriminate and protect against anything that may be harmful, absorb and integrate anything that supports your integrity and viability, and eliminate anything that doesn't serve to help you function at your best.

Eliminating, Integrating, and Nurturing

RELEASING AND HEALING: I invite you to go back to what you have written down during the examining exercise and ask yourself these questions:

> Is this story even true?
>
> Is it true that _____ (fill in)?
>
> What are the positive takeaways from this memory?
>
> What is positive about me? What are my virtues, victories, and values?

When you have come up with your three "Vs," choose one that resonates most deeply and positively with you and do the following:

PERFECT AS I AM MEDITATION

Breathe in for three counts, breathe out for five. Empty the mind (three cycles).

Breathe in for three, breathe out for five. Empty the heart (three cycles).

Breathe in for three, breathe out for five. Empty the digestive system of any negativity and let the flow of your breath move from your nose and mouth all the way down and out through the base of your spine (three cycles).

Bring your awareness to your solar plexus (stomach area) and breathe in for three, breathe out for five. Say to yourself "breathing in peace" on the inhale and "and harmony" on the exhale (five cycles).

Then as you breathe in and out, repeat these words with every cycle of breath, "I am perfect as I am and _____" (fill in your chosen virtue, value, or victory).

Do this as long as you wish and as often as you need to.

LOVE ON THE INSIDE AND OUTSIDE: Just like having a balanced ecosystem living within your gut, you want to work on having balanced loving in your own life. You are not meant to be an isolated being, just like those little friendly bacteria. Dr. Michael Gershon, author of *The Second Brain* and chairman of the department of anatomy and cell biology at Columbia University, has determined that oxytocin, the love hormone, very much influences the digestive system. In a 2010 study, Gershon found that oxytocin reduces gastrointestinal inflammation and improves gut motility.[3] This means bringing more love into your life:

- Fall in love with your life. Feel lucky. Rather than complaining about what you don't have or why you may be a "victim," choose instead to see the silver lining and realize that you "get to" do something, rather than "have to."

- Spend time out in nature, connecting to something vast and beautiful.

- Join a group. This could be a support group, spiritual group, or same-interest group. Finding people who share your interests enables you to feel less alone.

- Volunteer. When you do good for others, it feels good and also raises your oxytocin levels.

- Hug often and consider bodywork. Simple hugs and relaxing massages can also raise oxytocin levels. Touching reminds you that you are not alone.

- Choose to nourish yourself and your life *always*. Ask yourself before eating a certain food, engaging in a particular activity, or getting caught up in a negative thought or criticism: "How does this support me in being at my best, to flourish, grow, and be happy and healthy?"

DESTRESSING AND DIGESTING: High levels of stress shut down the digestive system in the variety of ways you have now learned about. You also now know that there are many ways to manage your stress levels, whether you develop a meditation practice, work through your emotions and practice cognitive restructuring, exercise, spend time out in nature, or talk to friends or a therapist.

In addition, you want to learn how to use food to be healthy, not to avoid feeling stress. Hectic lifestyles cause most people to eat on the go, quickly, without thinking or noticing what is going down. Many people use food for comfort, rather than fuel, which increases the stress response rather than lowering it. If you want to learn to change this habit, you can start eating mindfully:

- Appreciate the food on your plate—colors, smells, where it comes from, how lucky you are that you are about to be nourished, and so on.

- Choose a small bite, appreciate it, and when you place it in your mouth, notice everything about the taste and feeling. Chew slowly and thoroughly as you do so.

- When you swallow, once again think how lucky you are to be getting nourished.

- Take a few nice and slow breaths before the next bite.

- Stop when you notice that you feel full.

- Appreciate again.

Eating mindfully will help elicit the relaxation response, improve blood flow to the gut, improve breakdown, digestion, and absorption of food (especially if you really chew), and help put you in a place of appreciation rather than misery. In addition, you will likely find that you eat less and better and have an easier time maintaining a healthy weight.

Supporting Your Integrity and Viability

FUELING THE GUT: I want to emphasize *again* that it is important to start looking at food as fuel rather than as an outlet for comfort. Food, though it can still be comforting, can be ingested with the notion of nourishment in mind—something that supports you to be at your best, happiest, and healthiest.

You may be wondering what could be left for you to learn about healthy eating when you have read so much already. The goal in this section is to understand your digestive system, how your body uses and is affected by food. Sweets, baked goods, fatty foods, alcohol, excessive caffeine, a lot of dairy, or anything processed wreaks havoc on the digestive system, for example. In contrast, foods that are high in density and quality provide the natural vitamins and antioxidants your body needs and your digestive system requires for healthy functioning. This is what you need to know.

Stay *hydrated*. Fluid is absolutely necessary for digestion and absorption. Normally, you want to consume about half your body weight in ounces of water. So if you weigh 150 pounds, you want to drink 75 ounces of water throughout your day.

Before you start learning about which foods are best, know that no food gives you the nutrition you need if you do not *chew* it thoroughly first. The digestive juices in your saliva are key to getting the food into smaller particles, so that the nutrients are then accessible. How many times do you chew? Eat smaller portions at more frequent intervals and chew food to a pulp. Try counting to forty!

Do eat *protein*. Lean meat and eggs are easier for the gastrointestinal system to digest than processed meat and most fats. Some studies suggest that a diet high in red meat can increase your risk of colon cancer, though there is some debate as to the exact mechanism that leads to cancer.[4] To avoid this problem, if you do choose to eat red meat, keep your portion sizes small, go for the grass-fed lean meats, alternate with protein from other sources, such as legumes, healthy grains, and fish, and balance your plate with plenty of fruits and vegetables to provide antioxidants. Avoid processed meat; according to recent studies, such meats are linked to colon cancer due to the increased carcinogen content.[5]

Do eat *healthy fats*. Healthy fats are important for promoting healthy functioning of the digestive system (including the pancreas, liver, and gallbladder), reducing inflammation, improving heart health, weight control, regularity of bowel movements, and absorption of other nutrients such as antioxidants and fat-soluble vitamins like vitamin A. One good example is cod liver oil, which you probably know of as a good treatment to cleanse the gut and move bowels; but this oil is also high in vitamins A and D, and as I have mentioned before, vitamin D may be critically important in preventing the development of autoimmune conditions, including those of the gastrointestinal tract.[6]

You want to avoid hydrogenated oils, or oils that are liquid but become solid at room temperature. Also known as trans fats, these fats are hard on your gastrointestinal tract, difficult to digest, and associated with the variety of health problems you have already heard of, including high cholesterol and colon cancer. Hydrogenated fats are very bulky, requiring breakdown and then reformatting into particles that can be carried in the lymphatic system and then stored in fat cells to be utilized later. Can you understand now how the weight can build up, not to mention that you are feeding fat cells that can trigger your inflammatory response on their own?

Olive oil, a monounsaturated fat, safflower oil, a polyunsaturated fat, and coconut oil, a healthy saturated fat are examples of better oil choices that can lower cholesterol and inflammation and help with weight control. Coconut oil, in fact, because it is a medium-chain fatty acid, is broken down directly and taken to the liver to be used for fuel. Good fats include those you get from avocados, fatty fish, and nuts like almonds or walnuts.

When you shop, avoid the inside isles of the grocery store, keeping to the periphery where all the fresh and natural foods are located.

Fortify with *grains* and *fiber*. Fiber promotes digestive health by promoting regular bowel movements, helping you rid your body of waste. According to current studies, diets high in fiber are related to a lower risk of colon cancer.[7] In general, as I mentioned before, I recommend trying to keep your grain intake to the size of the palm of your hand and choosing to get more of your fiber from other complex carbohydrates, like broccoli, cauliflower, onions, leafy greens, berries, and other fruits; my two favorites (which happen to be great sources of fiber) are sweet potatoes and avocados.

Studies report an increasing number of gluten-sensitive people worldwide.[8] I have found in my clinical practice that the majority of my patients have some kind of gluten sensitivity, meaning their physical (not just digestive) and psychological symptoms are worse when they have a diet high in barley, rye, wheat, and other foods containing gluten—most processed foods like cookies, ketchup, salad dressing, and so on. Symptoms associated with sensitivity can range from bloating and heartburn to joint aches, fatigue, and depression. There are a variety of gluten-free grains that provide the body with fiber, minerals, vitamins, and protein necessary for healthy digestion and elimination. Some of them are oats, teff, millet, quinoa, and amaranth.

Restore the gut's ecosystem with *probiotics* and *prebiotics*. A healthy gut means having trillions of good bacteria living, digesting, absorbing, and promoting a healthy immune system. Eating processed and fast foods, living with a high level of stress and little sleep, or taking multiple rounds of antibiotics can result in the loss of this microflora and an imbalance or disharmony in the natural gut world, allowing disease-causing bacteria to thrive, inflammation to abound, and absorption of needed nutrients to remain poor. You therefore want to increase your intake of food groups that contain live cultures of such bacteria as *Lactobacillus* and *Bifidobacterium* as well as the foods that help feed them.

Yogurt that is made with "live" or "active" cultures is best, but you want to watch out for the amount of sugar that has been added. Go for unsweetened yogurt. You can add flax (for more fiber and antioxidants), berries, or honey, which also help the good bacteria thrive. Other foods that help the natural flora of your gut include onions, garlic, leeks, legumes, asparagus, and artichokes. Fermented foods are those that have been "cultured" and therefore also support the good bacteria. These include pickles, sauerkraut, tempeh, kefir, and miso.

Protect and heal with *antioxidants*. If you recall, your gut makes up a large part of your defense system against disease and pathogens through its physical barrier, its ecosystem (friendly bacteria), and the immune cells that live there. Your gut is constantly being invaded by the outside world, so if you do not ingest gut-friendly foods, damage and oxidative stress can occur. When damage occurs, you can be prone to developing a host of allergies, as your immune system becomes over-active, as well as other inflammatory problems affecting every part of your body. A good way to protect your gut, therefore, is by making sure you consume foods that are rich in antioxidants, like colorful fruits and vegetables (kale, raspberries, string beans, sweet potatoes, avocado, spinach, apples, and cantaloupe). Cherries, blueberries, tomatoes, and squash, for example, are high in antioxidants and may protect against inflammatory damage in the gut.

Consider *supplements*. If you have any gastrointestinal symptoms, have difficulty digesting many vegetables or fruits, sources of healthy fats, or fermented foods, you may want to supplement. Keep in mind that not all supplements are alike. You will need to check the labels and ask your health-care provider if they are safe for you, especially if you already have food allergies. In general, supplements that can boost your digestive health include probiotics, vitamin D, omega-3 fish oils, and digestive enzymes. You have already read about vitamin D and omega-3 fish oils, so I will focus here on probiotics and digestive enzymes.

A 2011 Agency for Healthcare Research and Quality assessment of the safety of probiotics concluded that the current evidence does not suggest a widespread risk of negative side effects associated with probiotics.[9] Probiotic supplementation has been found to support treatment of a variety of problems including diarrhea, especially after antibiotic use, inflammatory bowel disease, and symptoms associated with irritable bowel syndrome.[10] In general, friendly bacteria include *Bifidobacterium lactis* HN019 and Bb–12 (found in many yogurts), *Lactobacillus* (*L.*) *reuteri, L. rhamnosus, L. casei, L. acidophilus,* and *S. boulardii.* You want to check the label to ensure the full name of the bacteria is listed, and usually a variety of bacteria are better than one, matching the ecosystem in your gut.

Preliminary studies show that provision of digestive enzymes may support treatment of irritable bowel syndrome, heartburn, and celiac disease and may improve digestion.[11] Types of enzymes include hydrochloric acid, bromelain, lipase, lactase, and papain.

MOVING YOUR BODY GENTLY: Evidence suggests that low-intensity exercise may have protective effects on the gastrointestinal tract. There is strong evidence that the risk of colon cancer can be reduced by up to 50 percent with less but promising evidence for constipation, diverticulosis, bleeding, gallstones, and inflammatory bowel disease, though the underlying mechanisms are not fully understood.[12] For this reason, you want to incorporate regular gentle forms of exercise that advocate movement without too much stress, like certain forms of yoga, tai chi, and mindful walking.

SUPPORT, LOVE, AND JOY IN THE EATING ENVIRONMENT: As you have learned already, social support is good for your health and well-being. What better time to socialize than during mealtime? As the pace of our lives speeds up, many of us tend to eat on the run, in the car, and often alone, none of which supports our health and well-being. Individuals who eat with others are more likely to eat more slowly, make healthier food choices, and make mealtime more meaningful as an opportunity for sharing. Home-cooked meals also tend to be more nutritious. Studies show that adolescents who have regular family mealtimes are less likely to develop substance abuse problems.[13] This tells us that aside from the benefits of healthy nutrition, the togetherness of mealtime may provide you with the support and love you crave, so that you do not seek relief or comfort in maladaptive habits. With love comes oxytocin, which studies show is beneficial for gastrointestinal health.[14] So eat with others, be merry, and be happy and healthy!

CHAPTER EIGHT

The Musculoskeletal System

Move It or Lose It

There is more wisdom in your body than
in your deepest philosophy.

—FRIEDRICH NIETZSCHE

n my early forties, my joints ached every morning as I rose out of bed.
"I'm too young for this," I thought to myself. "I need to get stronger, physically. But what is the best way, when my back pain always seems to get in the way of really exercising?"

I closed my eyes and asked my lower back that very same question.

"Ha!" I heard a voice say. "You are so out of shape, of course your back hurts all of the time. This is what you need to do. . . ."

I then had a vision of being a female Tarzan, swinging on a rope, running as fast as a horse, and leaping from trees like a hawk in flight. When I landed back on the earth, I became a gentle female warrior, practicing martial-art movements. I felt a true sense of inner peace, because I had mastered the spiritual, mental, and physical realms of my existence.

A gentle warrior? Possibly. But a female Tarzan? Now that was laughable. I did understand in that moment, however, that I had spent many years honing my intellectual, mental, and spiritual abilities, but I had not paid much attention to my physical strength. My vision showed me that I could be a strong, resilient woman who had the capability of moving beyond human limitations not only spiritually, but physically, like flying from tree to tree and running like the wind, that it was time to cultivate a strong musculoskeletal system that could function as protection and support, so my life force could truly flourish.

Soon after this vision, I was introduced to CrossFit. Created by Greg Glassman in the 1980s, CrossFit is designed as a general physical preparedness program optimizing physical competence, improving cardiovascular and respiratory endurance, stamina, strength, flexibility, power, speed, coordination, agility, balance, and accuracy. The program uses weights, one's own body weight and flexibility, and the outdoors.

Initially, I was scared, and the program was hard, but I stuck with it. And now, in my late forties, I am in the best shape of my life. My core is solid, and I have more strength, agility, mobility, and flexibility than people who are twenty years younger. Not that I am swinging in trees every day (though I have been known to do so on occasion). But I am doing pull-ups and gymnastics moves that I couldn't even do as a teenager. What's more, I'm tougher. Challenges in life neither deter me nor scare me from pushing forward, and I have the energy to do it.

I am not sure why it took me so long to figure out that physical health is not just the physical health of your internal organs or your mental acuity. Your body is the vessel that allows you to be here on this earth. If your musculoskeletal system is not strong and agile, it is difficult to also be mentally, emotionally, and spiritually strong. Your mind, body, and spirit are one unit, and I, for one, had often forgotten this fact, because I had spent so much time poring over books or sitting in cars or in front of a computer. I had forgotten that we were meant to coexist with nature, running, walking, lifting, climbing, squatting, and jumping. I had lost touch with the notion that we need a physical shell that is both strong and protective, agile and full of robust energy, so that we can keep moving through life.

Indeed, I think many of us take the human musculoskeletal system for granted and forget how amazing it actually is that we are able to walk upright on two limbs. Your skeletal system includes bones, ligaments, connective tissue, and cartilage, all of which support the weight of the body and protect the delicate internal organs. With the muscles, the skeleton works to maintain and produce controlled movements and body position, so that as muscles contract and relax, push and pull, you are able to walk, run, sit, squat, lift, or lie down. This system enables many functions that allow you to survive, including mobility, flexibility, and stability as well as protection, support, and nourishment.

In this chapter, you will learn how to regain or enhance the POWER of your musculoskeletal system, as you:

- Press the PAUSE button and become acquainted with the anatomy and functions of the musculoskeletal system.

- OPTIMIZE your awareness of what can go wrong with your muscles and bones, the signs and symptoms to watch out for that tell you to get medical help, and what you can learn from wisdom traditions and their view of the musculoskeletal system and its functions.

- Discover how your muscles, joints, and bones may be speaking to you as you WITNESS your physiology through guided exercises.

- EXAMINE the emotions and beliefs that may be keeping you from being flexible, balanced, strong, and mobile.

- Develop the tools that will enable you to RELEASE negative habits and beliefs that are keeping you stiff and immobile, RELIEVE your aches and pains, and RESTORE your musculo-skeletal system to optimal shape.

PAUSE and OPTIMIZE Your Awareness of Your Musculoskeletal System

Anatomy and Functions

A living, breathing system, the musculoskeletal system is composed of bones, muscles, ligaments, tendons, cartilage, and fascia that create an intricate network with your brain, heart, and immune system.

Your skeletal system provides you with support, stability, and protection. To begin, you have 206 bones in your body, though you start as an infant with 270 (some fuse as you grow). This network of bones is called an endoskeleton, meaning that the frame that gives you support is inside the shell of soft tissue, as opposed to outside, like that of a crustacean. Since you will learn about the vertebrae in your spine in the next chapter, here I will focus on the appendicular skeleton, or the bones in the rest of the body, arms, and legs, which enable you to walk, run, and move as well as protect major organs like the heart, lungs, digestive tract, and reproductive organs.

Your bones are made out of the structural protein collagen and such minerals as calcium, sodium, and phosphorous. The calcium content of your bones, which is very much affected by your vitamin D levels and calcium intake, determines how hard they are. Your bones are in a continuous process of reshaping and remodeling throughout your lifetime, so that your skeleton can maintain a normal bone mass and be able to respond to mechanical forces. This process is dependent on the functioning of hormones, like parathyroid hormone, that respond to changes in blood calcium and phosphorus. When the circulating calcium or phosphorous levels in the bloodstream are low, meaning these minerals are in short supply, these hormones will pull out these minerals from the bone. If these withdrawals occur too frequently, the bones will eventually weaken. Intestinal calcium and phosphorus absorption is regulated by vitamin D, and a deficiency of this vitamin can not only cause levels of calcium and phosphorous to be low, but also stimulate the parathyroid hormone, resulting in more "withdrawals."

Your bones have an outer hard layer called compact bone and a less dense layer called cancellous bone. The outside layer is made up of hard osteon, which has nerves and blood vessels running through the center that serves to nourish and protect the bone and bone marrow. The bone marrow is found within the cancellous bone, where blood cells are produced.

Ligaments connect bones to bones and help support and stabilize the skeleton in place, especially with movement. Continuous sheets of thin tissue, or fascia, surround and fuse with your bones, muscles, nerves, blood vessels, tendons, and internal organs throughout the entire body, allowing the muscles to work with varying intensity, so that surrounding structures, like your organs, are protected from harm.

The bones meet one another at joints, which are held in place by muscles and ligaments. Joints usually enable varying degrees of mobility, depending upon where they are. Synovial joints are those found in the hips, elbows, fingers, and knees and are given this name because they have a synovial lining that releases fluid to keep the joints lubricated. The ends of the bones are covered by slippery and smooth material called articular cartilage, which also allows the joints to move with little friction. A fibrous capsule keeps the joint in place.

Joints are categorized into types, based on the kind of mobility they allow you. For instance, the ball and socket allows movement in several directions and is found in the shoulder joint, between the humerus and scapula, and in the hip joint, between the femur and the hipbone. Your knee joint, on the other hand, only allows movement in a single direction and is called a hinge joint. Your wrists and ankles have pivot joints that allow more mobility than your knee, but less than your shoulders or hips. The joint with the least mobility is the one that connects your skull to your spine.

Your muscles cover and connect your bones and are intricately connected to your brain and your nervous system, so that you can actually move. Attached to the bones via tendons, the muscles contract and relax, pulling your bones to and fro. When you decide you want to move, motor neurons, or nerve cells that control movement, in the brain send an electrical signal through the spinal cord and nervous system to the muscles. The neurons in the nervous system transmit a signal, known as an action potential, to individual muscle fibers through a release of energy in the form of adenosine triphosphate, or ATP. The release of ATP causes the muscles to shorten and contract, pulling on the connective tissue and drawing the bone into movement. The kind of movement that occurs will depend on the specific muscle that contracts around the designated joint—like bending at the knees or pronating of the wrists. The signal to relax enables the muscle opposing the contracted muscle to extend the movable bone back to its original position.

If you really think about how your body manages to move in this way, it is really quite fascinating. My hope is that a little bit of this understanding will go a longer way in encouraging you not to take this intricate system for granted.

What Can Go Wrong?

Bones can weaken or break; joints can become inflamed, dislocated, full of fluid, or degenerated. Muscles can become weak or tight, and neurons can misfire or be unable to fire. Weak muscles in your right leg will lead to more pressure and joint damage in your left leg. The weakness or imbalance can also strain connective tissue and joints, leading to more damage of the bone. Drying up of the fluid in your joints will lead to friction, poor mobility, and eventually bone damage as well. One part affects the others. As the system breaks down, you can lose mobility, flexibility, and even the ability to stand upright and move—and those are just the physical complications.

Problems affecting the musculoskeletal system usually lead to pain and discomfort and can result in a disruption in everyday activities, including sitting, standing, or finding a comfortable position to sleep in. The longer the problems continue, the higher the chances that other parts of the body will be negatively affected or that bone damage may occur. Any one of the joints is susceptible, including the neck, spine, hips, knees, elbows, shoulders, wrists, hands, and feet, and symptoms can include recurrent pain, stiffness, dull aches, muscle spasm pains, weakness, and swelling.

The most common musculoskeletal problems include:

- Fibromyalgia: A syndrome causing pain and tenderness in various parts of the body, including muscles, joints, tendons, and other soft tissues.

- Osteoarthritis: Also known as degenerative joint disease, the most common type of problem affecting joints. It is usually due to aging and wear and tear. Normally this occurs because of the wearing away of the cartilage, which causes the bones to rub together. Swelling, pain, stiffness, and weakening of tendons and muscles can occur.

- Rheumatoid Arthritis: An autoimmune disorder affecting all joints that may also affect internal organs over time.

- Bursitis: A condition that occurs when the fluid-filled sac that acts as a cushion between the joints, muscles, and tendons gets inflamed, irritated, and swollen.

- Tendonitis: A condition that occurs when there is inflammation, irritation, or swelling of a tendon, commonly affecting such areas as the Achilles heel, shoulder (rotator cuff), elbow (tennis elbow), or wrist.

- Gout: A type of arthritis or inflammation of the joints caused by a buildup of uric acid in the blood. Usually only one joint is affected, often the big toe.

- Repetitive Strain Injury: A condition in which overuse puts too much stress or strain on the same part of the body too many times, which results in inflammation, swelling, muscle strain, or damage.

- Osteomyelitis: Infection of the bone that may occur after some sort of trauma.

- Osteoporosis: A condition in which bones become weak, brittle, thin, and spongy, so that they can break easily. It usually occurs with aging, steroid use, or use of other medications like warfarin.

Causes and Risk Factors

As a general rule, musculoskeletal conditions usually have diverse causes and are typically influenced by age, type of occupation, lifestyle behaviors, and the nature, frequency, and intensity of a physical activity. For instance, running for long distances can frequently lead to severe wear and tear on the knees. Heavy lifting or sitting for long periods in the same position may add to degeneration of the back. Osteoarthritis, bursitis, and tendonitis can all occur with overuse or injury or even from being overweight.

Conditions like fibromyalgia have been linked to poor sleep, fatigue, headaches, depression, and a history of emotional or physical trauma.[1] In my clinical experience, every patient who has come in with a diagnosis of "fibromyalgia" has had a long-standing history of poor sleep or sleep deprivation. The connection between these two conditions is unclear, but is likely partially due to chronic inflammation, stress, and the inability of the muscles to fully relax as they normally do during deep sleep.

Statistically, women between the ages of twenty and fifty are more likely to get fibromyalgia, though it is my clinical experience the male-female distribution has been about equal. Women are also more likely to get rheumatoid arthritis, though it can occur at any age and may be linked to changes in genetic patterns, hormones, or infections.[2] Gout, on the other hand, is more common in men and in individuals who drink a lot of alcohol. Gout has also been linked to other medical conditions, including diabetes, obesity, high cholesterol, kidney disease, and certain medications.[3]

Musculoskeletal conditions often have neither a gender preference nor a genetic basis. They simply occur because of the wear and tear that comes with the aging process.

The Painful Facts

- Musculoskeletal disorders are the leading cause of disability in the United States.

- In people over fifty years of age in developed countries, musculoskeletal disorders account for more than 50 percent of all chronic conditions.

- In 2005, musculoskeletal conditions were reported by 107.67 million adults in the United States, representing nearly one in two persons age eighteen and older.

- For the years 2004–2006, for musculoskeletal conditions, the sum of the direct expenditures in health-care costs and the indirect expenditures in lost wages has been estimated to be $950 billion annually, or 7.4 percent of the national gross domestic product.[4]

Red Flags That Signal You Should Seek Medical Attention

Though most conditions are mild and often heal on their own, for some it is best to seek medical advice or attention:

- An injury, for which a radiographic assessment is necessary.

- An obvious fracture or dislocation, especially an open fracture. Dislocations should be reduced immediately. If there seems to be a lack of circulation in the affected limb, this is an emergency, as blood supply may be compromised.

- Severe, ongoing pain that is not relieved with regular pain medications like acetaminophen or ibuprofen.

- Pain that seems to be coming from the abdomen or chest.

- Swelling of the lower leg and pain in the calf (can indicate a clot in the vein).

- Some sort of nerve compromise like tingling, numbness, weakness, or searing pain that travels down the leg, down the arm, or from one location to the next.

- A chronic compartment syndrome: aching, burning, tightness, tingling/numbness, or weakness, usually in a limb, which gets worse with exercise and often gets better slightly after thirty minutes of stopping exercise. Chronic compartment syndrome, which can also occur acutely after trauma and is a medical emergency, involves swelling of the myofascial compartment of the limb, leading to compromised circulation to the affected muscles. Usually pain upon stretching is excruciating and seems to be much worse than on first examination.

- A joint that is swollen, red, hot/warm or tender to the touch, which can indicate a septic or infected joint. Pain is usually constant and throbbing, keeping individuals awake at night and severely limiting mobility. This is also a medical emergency.

- Nerve compression with a back injury or a history of back problems, especially if accompanied by weakness, loss of sensation, impotence, or loss of anal tone, whereby the stool cannot be held in.[5]

Note: Some symptoms seem musculoskeletal in nature, but are actually symptoms that originate from your heart, lungs, or abdomen, for example. Watch out for other symptoms like shortness of breath, a change (up or down) of blood pressure, chest pain that radiates down your arm or up your jaw, or severe mid-back pain.

Remember, these conditions are treatable by allopathic medicine. Do not hesitate to go and have the appropriate evaluation and treatment. Pay attention to what your body needs, especially when it is screaming.

What Wisdom Traditions Say About Bones, Muscles, and Joints

Wisdom traditions view movement as essential to life. When the musculoskeletal system is healthy, we are able to move through life with ease and flow. When unhealthy, we tend to get stuck, and our bodies become sore and stiff. Having a supple body accordingly reflects a supple and open attitude toward life, while a strong body represents solid core beliefs, a sense of purpose, and the constitution to withstand life's challenges. In other words, when the musculoskeletal system is thriving, our mobility; flexibility; sense of feeling protected, supported, and nourished; and ability to powerfully move through the world are booming too.

Traditional Chinese medicine sees the bones, muscles, and joints coexisting like the elements of nature. The muscles, for instance, fall under the element of "wood," which is involved in such physical aspects as extension, germination or growth, movement, and strength and such mental aspects as self-assertion, planning, decision making, and forceful action. The bones are representative of the "water" element, which is aligned with support, conservation of resources, adaptability, persistence, determination, and courage. The joints, because they are open cavities of space like the lungs, are connected to the element of "metal," which, as you may recall, is connected to taking in and letting go, appreciation versus grief, searching for purity and truth, inspiration, and self-respect.

According to traditional Chinese medicine, then, if you were having a problem with your joints or muscles, you might also be struggling with your sense of purpose or your rightful place in life. You may be feeling frustrated, stuck, unhappy, unsupported, or lost. You may also tend to hold back, lack assertiveness or confidence, be critical or judgmental, or be too disciplined or worried to make a move. Perhaps you are scared to make changes or you are grieving the loss of a loved one.

Thoughts, beliefs, and emotions can thus be intertwined with musculoskeletal issues. Tensing muscles can point to frustration, stagnation, and anger. Problems with the joints, like problems with the lungs, may be pointing toward issues related to loss, beating oneself up (especially in the case of an autoimmune disorder), or lack of self-confidence.

I have found that my patients learn a lot about themselves, their beliefs, their desires—especially how they truly relate to challenging experiences—when they examine their musculoskeletal symptoms more closely.

At forty years old, Alice reported that she had been extremely healthy until injuring her left shoulder two years earlier. She had had surgery and physical therapy on the shoulder eight months before seeing me. The pain had improved, only to worsen again four months later. To make matters worse, her right hip started hurting too. The pain became so bad that it disturbed her sleep, so that she now also found herself sleep deprived and anxious. She felt frustrated that she was not healing, despite having gone to physical therapy, cognitive behavioral therapy, and doing everything else that she was told to do. Nothing was helping except for strong doses of ibuprofen, which were irritating her stomach. Alice complained of being constantly tired, anxious, and on the brink of despair. She was becoming dependent on her mother and husband and simply hated it.

I asked Alice about the injury and when the pain seemed to get worse. She told me she had initially hurt her shoulder during a fall while skiing. Surgery had revealed no tears, but some calcium deposits had been removed. She went to physical therapy after that for a few months and took pain medication, but because it was difficult to lie flat in a bed, she had to sleep in an easy chair, which meant she hardly ever got a good night's sleep. In addition, she started having problems with her left hip, which was affecting her mobility throughout the day.

I asked Alice if anything significant or stressful had happened in addition to these problems during this time.

Alice's initial reaction was to say no, but then she held her breath, let out a big exhale, and said, "Actually, yes. My grandmother died a few months before. She was a big part of my life." Alice's eyes began to tear as she explained that she had been an only child and when her father had taken ill when Alice was nine years old, her grandmother became her other caretaker.

After giving Alice some time to begin to develop her own connection between the loss and the injury, I asked her to close her eyes, focus on her left shoulder, and describe to me what she felt, to see if the pain she experienced had an origination point—for instance, whether it came from the shoulder itself, the neck, the back, or the chest.

This is what Alice told me: "It feels like it is coming from my heart. I feel an ache and a tightness. I feel sad."

"Why do you feel sad, Alice? Where does this sadness come from? See how far back the sadness takes you." I said.

"I was twelve years old. My boyfriend broke up with me. I was devastated and cried for a long time. My mom tried to comfort me, but she wasn't around enough. She felt bad. My grandmother tried to console me, but my grandfather was sick then too. I felt very rejected and insecure. It wasn't fair. I never wanted to feel this way again," Alice continued.

"Did you feel this way again, Alice?"

"Yes. When my father's sister died, when I broke up with my college boyfriend, and again when my grandmother died."

"Alice," I said, "Can you ask your shoulder if there is a connection between your pain and all these losses?"

"I just feel scared. I am scared to be left alone with nothing."

"Why would you be left alone? Are you not happy in your marriage, your job, or your life?"

"No, I am not happy. I feel stuck in my job and my marriage. I have security, but no freedom, but I am too scared to leave. I'm stuck."

At this point, Alice and I discussed her fear of loss and abandonment that resulted in her choosing security over freedom and the exploration of her own identity. Perhaps, I theorized, her muscles were bracing for being left alone, rejected, or abandoned again. Perhaps her feeling of being alone exacerbated her inability to sleep. Most likely, her pain, her inability to sleep, and her anxiety were a combination of physical, emotional, and spiritual issues that were asking to be taken care of.

Alice's treatment plan included meditation and healing exercises that helped her address and deal with feelings of loss and grief as well as stretching exercises that enabled her to feel more grounded, supported, and aligned. We worked on reestablishing a support network within her friends and family, examining her true desires and life purpose, the skills she valued and the work possibilities she could explore. I also introduced an exercise plan that would enable her to resume mobility and strength. Alice changed her diet so that she ate fewer inflammatory foods, and she added in omega-3 fish oils, which would help with inflammation and mood. She also started couple's counseling with her husband to see if spice and direction could be brought back into their marriage.

Within seven months, Alice was pain free and feeling better than ever. She found a new job, new friends, new hobbies, and, most important, she rediscovered happiness.

Deciphering What Science and Wisdom Traditions Say

When examining what messages your body may be holding and why, keep in mind the functions of the musculoskeletal system: mobility, flexibility, and movement as well as protection, support, stability, and nourishment. For instance, a major role of this system is to provide structure and framework to support the body as it stands and moves on this earth. If your problems tend to be in your feet or knees, this could represent your own deep-seated beliefs about feeling supported or grounded in your life, since your feet and knees literally help you stand on the earth. If your muscles are continuously tense, perhaps you do not feel safe, supported, or strong enough within yourself, which may cause you to brace and protect what is on the inside from the outside.

When you were born, although you had close to three hundred bones, you did not possess the ability to stand upright or move from one position to another. You depended entirely on someone else. As you grew and developed, your bones began to fuse, your muscles developed strength, and your brain matured, so that your cerebral cortex and cerebellum could help you stay balanced, upright, and moving in the directions you chose to go. In addition, if you were being taken care of and loved, you had a strong supportive framework from which to develop and grow. Without such a framework, insecurity and lack of self-confidence in your own strengths and the ability to move forward could arise. Experiences of loss, neglect, criticism, or abuse could have led to feelings of fear and the need to constantly protect yourself from the unknown or push harder to get your needs met.

When observing your musculoskeletal system, think about the ways you may not feel supported, energized, or able to move beyond your fears. Think about your "weak spot" and why, of all places in your body, you are having difficulty there. Or perhaps you have been diagnosed with fibromyalgia, so your body tends to ache all over. You may want to examine how long it has been since you have had a restful sleep, what you may be scared of, how safe or supported you feel, and whether you believe that your needs will be met by others or the world within which you exist. I can personally tell you that when I addressed my fears about security or being supported, my back pain improved. When I added exercise and an anti-inflammatory diet, it virtually went away.

Why not give it a go?

WITNESS the Physiology of Your Musculoskeletal System

AWARENESS EXERCISE

Begin with the practice of emptying the mind.

Breathe in, breathe out. Empty the mind.

Bring your awareness to your feet. Notice how they feel touching the earth.

Notice where your weight falls with respect to your feet. Where is the pressure? What are your toes doing? Notice the connection between the toes and feet.

Notice the connection between your feet and ankles. Move your feet in circles slowly. Appreciate the mobility and what your toes, feet, and ankles enable you to do.

Move up your legs, noticing your calves and shins, up to your knees, again appreciating their purpose. Notice what you feel. Examine the joints. What do you feel?

Observe your muscles, joints, tendons, ligaments, your movement or ability to be coordinated as you move up your body, up your spine, and all the way up to the top of your head.

When you are done, focus on one or two joints (like your hips, shoulders, or knees) and notice any sensations that may come up for you with these images, thoughts, or scenarios:

I am going in the direction I want to be going in my life.

I feel frustrated and stuck.

I am not getting the support I need.

I am running a 5K race.

I am stuck in a wheelchair.

I am resentful that I am always left doing all the work.

I am not working in a job that represents my desires and likes.

I grieve a lost one.

Take as long as you wish to appreciate what you might feel and where, as you will have a chance to go deeper and better understand what lies beneath. You may wish to write down your experience in your journal, so that you can add to it later.

EXAMINE Your Deeper Emotions and Beliefs

First review the following statements and note how they cause you to feel, noticing which ones ring true or false. Then, write down what comes to mind as an answer.

Support, Protection, and Stability:

I am not good at asking for help.

I usually end up doing things myself.

I feel supported in most if not all ways by my partner to be the best I can be in my life.

I am often angry that I am not supported, appreciated, or recognized enough (at work, at home, in life, and so on).

I tend to distrust that I will have my needs met.

I am often angry that my needs are not met.

I am scared of rejection and being hurt.

Movement and Flexibility:

My life is moving in the direction I want to be going (or I lack a sense of direction).

I feel stuck in my situation (job, relationship, health issue, and so on).

I feel held back from doing what I want to do.

Something is irritating me or frustrating me, so that I feel I cannot fully express myself and have to hold back.

I am afraid to move forward or express myself more.

Provision and Rebuilding:

I am not sure what my purpose is.

I have a hard time giving my body time for rest. (I do not know what will happen if I rest.)

I often eat foods that do not nurture my life force.

I am often tired and have little energy to fight through the struggles in my life.

I often hold on to negative thoughts and feelings.

I have a hard time letting go.

GOING DEEPER EXERCISE

Choose one or more statements that provoked you the most, then take a few deep breaths, and close your eyes.

Breathe three more times fully and completely, then bring your awareness to the area of your body that seemed the most symptomatic to you during the witnessing exercise, repeat one or more of the statements, and see or feel what transpires.

Do you start feeling more or less tension?

Take your time and allow images, words, or thoughts to come forward.

Do you see anything? What image or thought comes up for you? Ask the thought, belief, image, or statement where it came from. Where did you learn it? When did you come up with it? What does it have to do with your body now?

When you are ready, write about your experience, adding it to your journal. Allow one thought to lead to the next without too much analysis or judgment, and see where it takes you.

As I mentioned, you want to pay attention not only to your answers, but also to your feelings—both physical and emotional—as Alice did.

RELEASE, RELIEVE, and RESTORE

Strengthening and healing the musculoskeletal system translates to being more vibrant and resilient in both body and mind. Your outlets of relief are focused on reducing rigidity, while improving flexibility and movement. They are also geared toward letting go of fears, working toward living your life with gusto and trust, and enhancing your sense of feeling safe and secure within yourself and your world, so that you move through life with more ease and can express yourself more energetically.

Support, Protection, and Stability

RELEASING: The purpose of this meditation is to enable you to let go of the story that became evident to you in the examination exercise. Is your story related to fear of loss, not being supported, or not having enough? Let it go, and instead focus on trusting that you can be supported to be free of your fears and able to move beyond your own expectations.

SUPPORTED AND FREE MEDITATION

Begin with the practice of emptying the mind. Breathe in deeply for three counts, then exhale for five counts. Release all the thoughts to the wind and to the earth. Do this for at least four cycles.

Bring your awareness to your spine (from the base of your skull to the base of the spine), to your entire back (all the muscles), ribs, and shoulders. Breathing in for three counts and out for five, empty the stress, strain, tension, or burdens you have been carrying that have been holding you back and stuck into the wind and into the earth. Do this for at least four cycles.

Bring your awareness to your chest and abdomen. Breathing in for three counts and out for five, release all tension, stress, strain or whatever has been holding you back from fully living, breathing, and expressing into the wind and into the earth. Do this for at least four cycles.

Do the same for both your arms and legs, fingers and toes.

You have released the stress and strain, so that now you can notice the support you actually do have. Notice the support your body has from the earth, wherever you lie.

Now notice the support the earth gives your feet as you imagine standing at the base of a mountain.

Breathe in the air. Feel the breeze against your skin. Listen to the birds flying in the sky. It is you and nature. Let nature and the earth guide you as you climb the mountain.

You are letting go of fears. You are moving forward with instinct and without questioning how or why.

You are climbing up the mountain with grace and ease. No fear. No judgment. Just moving.

You are at the top of the mountain. You stand tall. You can accomplish what you desire.

You spread your arms like wings and fly. You are free.

Repeat these words to yourself:

I am free.

I am free to fly.

I am free to express myself as I need to.

I am confident, strong, adaptable, adventurous, and joyous.

I am.

You slowly glide back down to earth. Your feet are firmly planted on the earth. You are supported.

I am supported.

I am supported to express myself as I need to.

I am confident, strong, adaptable, adventurous, and joyous.

I am.

SEEKING SUPPORT AND LETTING GO: Freedom to express yourself and move forward in life requires also feeling safe and secure in relation to others and within yourself. What will it take for you to let go of your toxic beliefs, lifestyle habits, and restrictions, so that you can be free to breathe and be you? Practicing the above meditation is helpful, but you want to build an external support structure within your life, people you can talk to, share with, or grow with. You can speak to a therapist, support group, religious community, or friends to help you. What will it be?

Support and letting go can also involve a healing touch. Your muscles and bones crave the structure, the oxytocin, and the relief you can get from a massage, adjustment, or whatever healing modality serves you best.

LIVING WITH PURPOSE: As you clear your mind and body of negative beliefs and fears that block you from moving forward in your life, you open up channels within you and your life for discovering who you really are and what your purpose can be. Your purpose can take a number of sizes and shapes—from healing the planet to raising healthy and open-minded children. Studies show that individuals who believe they have a purpose in life are healthier and live longer.[6] Feeling purposeful in your actions also helps you become more directed, engaged, and motivated to get up and go.

Whether you believe you know your purpose or not, you may want to add to your journal by writing about what is meaningful to you and how you would like to be able to bring more meaning into your life or the world. You may want to write about what has blocked you from doing so before and begin to make a list of small steps you can take toward your goal every week. For instance, maybe you feel your purpose is to cultivate good relationships and connections among the people you know. Write about why this is meaningful to you and what has prevented you from actively doing this with purpose, and make a plan to introduce one person to the next in a meaningful way every week.

Movement and Flexibility

TONING, STRENGTHENING, AND SWEATING: Your musculoskeletal system craves variability of movement, not sitting still for long hours or even performing the same activities over and over again. Variability is the key for adaptability and flexibility. This means being engaged in a variety of activities that include aerobic exercise and metabolic conditioning as well as resistance training, all mixed up so that your body is continuously surprised and rebuilding itself and its priorities.

The CDC recommends incorporating physical activity that includes aerobic conditioning, strength building, and balance training. The guidelines recommend at least 150 minutes a week of moderate physical exercise or 75 minutes of vigorous exercise (meaning you cannot carry on a conversation while exercising).[7] You want to remember that your body needs all kinds of movement, but so does your mind, as most individuals can easily get bored and drop their exercise routine. Varying your exercise routine will be helpful for not only improving your cardiovascular metabolism, strength, and flexibility, but also keeping you motivated. You can mix it up: alternate two to three days of shorter and more intense workouts that involve strength training with rest days and days when you perform low-intensity movement like walking, hiking, or taking a slow bike ride.

There is such a thing as excessive exercise, which can create more stress and damage for you than good. Strength-training workouts do not need to involve weights necessarily, as you can use your own body weight with movements such as push-ups, pull-ups, squats, or lunges. These types of exercises help you build lean muscle mass, strengthen your bones, and improve your metabolism.

The most important part of your exercise regimen should be that it is fun. If you are not enjoying yourself, you probably won't stick to it. These are some suggestions to make exercise more enjoyable, so that you will be more likely to keep it up, and an activity that helps you feel more supported:

- Find friends/exercise buddies or an exercise community.

- Do a variety of exercises that you enjoy, so that you do not get bored.

- Exercise outdoors, where, research shows, you are more likely to enjoy the workout and have less discomfort or fatigue.

- Do not set big goals for yourself. Exercise because you want to feel good.

- Be spontaneous and match your workout with your energy level. In other words, if you haven't slept well and are tired, do not engage in a high-intensity workout.

MEDITATION IN MOTION: Your goal is to move with ease in your life as well as to make your body move with ease. Practicing meditation while in motion enables you to stay present in your body and in your surroundings, while letting go of fears, stress, and strain. The result is better flexibility and mobility not only because you are becoming more relaxed and less tense, because you are stretching and loosening, but also because you are engaging. You can find many such exercises and a variety of techniques by working with practitioners who do yoga, tai chi, qi gong, or even Feldenkrais, a technique that helps you explore new movement patterns using gentle motion with directed attention.

Sample Week of Exercise

Day 1: A walk outdoors at a moderate pace with a friend for thirty minutes at 75 percent of your maximum heart rate.

Day 2: Strength training for twenty-five minutes using weights or your own body weight.

Day 3: Aerobics class, Zumba class, or a hike at a fast pace at intervals. You can walk at a moderate pace for a few minutes, then sprint for twenty seconds over a forty-five minute period.

Day 4: Active rest: walk your dog or someone else's dog, ride your bike, or stroll at a leisurely pace (at about 55 percent of your maximum heart rate) for an hour, as you enjoy the wonders of nature.

Day 5: Strength training for twenty-five minutes.

Day 6: A walk outdoors with a friend for thirty minutes at 75 percent of your maximum heart rate.

Day 7: Rest, or active rest as above.

Stretching as a general rule helps you warm up all your joints, muscles, and bones, work out kinks, and prevent stiffness. Stretching mindfully involves using your breath as you move, enabling gentle motion with directed attention. You can also walk mindfully.

Here is an exercise that brings walking and stretching mindfully together:

MINDFUL MOVEMENT IN NATURE

Begin by taking a slow walk in nature, being mindful of your breath while appreciating the beauty and wonder of the elements around you—the smell of the flowers, the blueness of the sky, or the variety of shapes and sizes of the leaves on the trees.

When you are ready, find a place to stand on the earth, perhaps barefoot, and recognize the connection your feet have with the earth.

Take a deep breath in and expand your chest so that your shoulders are rotating outwards (as if your scapulae are kissing), and when you exhale, allow your shoulders to roll back in. Your hands will follow as the shoulders rotate out and then back in.

Recognize your connection with the air.

Rotate your head to look to the left and hold it for two breaths, bring it back to center, and then look to the right for two breaths.

Recognize your connection with all of your surroundings.

Bend forward at the hips and bend your knees slightly as you place your hands with arms straight and locked above your knees. Breathe in and arch your back upward, like a cat or an upside-down "U." Then exhale and let your back fall back toward the earth.

Do this for three breath cycles and recognize your connection with all your internal organs, arms, and legs.

When you are ready, continue your slow, mindful walk through nature.

MOVING BEYOND LIMITS: You want to work on pushing yourself beyond your comfort zone, safely of course. What have you always wanted to try, but were too scared to do? Dance, paint, take a different route to work, sing out loud, take a class in something you always wanted to learn? Just do it! Moving beyond your limits does not have to occur just with physical exercise; it can apply to anything you do in your life. Do not let your fears create obstacles for you that leave you feeling stuck and unfulfilled. What will it be? Set a goal and go for it.

Provision and Rebuilding

NUTRIENTS FOR STAYING MOBILE: As you have learned thus far, a healthy nutrition plan involves eating foods that are anti-inflammatory, high in antioxidants, and full of healthy proteins, fats, vitamins, and minerals. The recommendations in this chapter will help you attain the desired goal of staying flexible, mobile, and pain free as well as help you maintain a healthy weight. The goal is to enable you to add foods to your diet that help motivate you to participate in physical activity, as they help reduce your perception of fatigue and therefore influence your mind-set to want to exercise and enjoy your experience.

Avoid foods that *slow you down*. As I have mentioned before, you want to focus on avoiding foods that are highly inflammatory, tax your metabolism, and prevent absorption of the vitamins and minerals you need. Such foods include breads, especially white breads, baked goods made with cornstarch, most dairy, fried foods, artificial sweeteners, beer, soda, and anything with high-fructose corn syrup.

Get your *vegetables and fruits* on! You can't go wrong eating more vegetables and fruits (in moderation), especially if you are choosing dark leafy greens for the many reasons you have read about thus far. Some studies have shown that a vegan diet that is also gluten free is beneficial for individuals with rheumatoid arthritis.[8] Other colorful dietary components, cherries, for example, have been shown to be helpful in reducing postexercise pain and muscle-cell damage and inflammation as well as a more rapid restoration of muscle strength.[9] Green leafy vegetables and other vegetables like beets have components like nitrates that enable better oxygenation and blood flow. Greens are also, of course, a good source of magnesium, important for both muscle and bone function and strength.

Keep up your stamina with *healthy grains*. Grains are a good source of complex carbohydrates, fiber, minerals, vitamins, and antioxidants. Your muscles need glycogen (from glucose), which gives them more energy and helps you stay active longer. Wheat germ, for example, contains octacosanol, which helps with muscle oxygenation and the prevention of strains or injury. Oats, a good alternative to grains with gluten, are a good source of silicon, which helps strengthen connective tissue. If you notice that you have a tendency to feel achy or have poor recovery after exercise, you may also want to try a gluten-free diet, even if you have never been diagnosed with a sensitivity. Try eating only grains like millet, quinoa, brown rice, buckwheat, sorghum, amaranth, or teff.

Use *fats* to stay flexible. Foods rich in good fats, like omega-3 fatty acids, alpha-linolenic acid, and linolenic acid, can help with elasticity and muscle flexibility and to reduce inflammation.[10] You can get these benefits from flaxseed, olive oil, avocados, fatty fish, algae, and hemp. For example, fish intake has been linked to improved muscle strength and physical performance.[11]

Pump up your *muscle and bone mass*. Protein enables you to maintain adequate bone and muscle health. Good sources come from grass-fed meats, fish, grains (like quinoa, brown rice, and amaranth), vegetables (like peas), and plants (like hemp), nuts, legumes, and soy and milk products. Fish are also a good source of vitamin D, which, as you learned, is important for bone health and calcium absorption. If you suffer from inflammatory joint problems, like rheumatoid arthritis, you may want to limit the majority of your protein to vegetables, grains, or plants and nuts, as animal sources of protein may lead to more pain for some individuals.[12]

Drink up (water!). Every system of your body needs water. Recommendations for the daily amount of water you should drink vary, because the amount depends on your existing health condition, what you eat, and how much activity you engage in, among other factors. The Institute of Medicine determined that an adequate intake for men is roughly 3 liters (about 13 cups) of total beverages a day. The adequate intake for women is 2.2 liters (about 9 cups) of total beverages a day.[13] In general, as I mentioned before, you can aim to drink about half your body weight in ounces a day.

Perhaps *supplements* are in order. If you are unable to get your nutrition through your diet or are an athlete in training, many of these nutritional needs can be met with supplements. I will not go into depth on supplements, but I do find eggshell membrane to be highly effective for supporting joint health, along with glucosamine and chondroitin. A recent study shows promise that eggshell membrane is effective and safe for treating pain and inflexibility associated with joint and connective tissue disorders.[14] Of course, check with your health-care provider for interactions or contraindications as necessary. Dosages are product dependent.

DESTRESSING AND RESTING: This is most likely an obvious one for you. Pay attention to your stress levels as you go through your day. Practice mindfulness and your breathing exercises. Meet with a therapist, talk to friends, take relaxing baths—whatever it takes to help you with your stress reduction.

Your muscles need to know that they can let go and relax now and then. Otherwise they forget how to. That is why it is so important to get good and restful sleep. It is rare for individuals to get fibromyalgia if they actually get adequate sleep. If sleep is an issue for you, you may want to work with your health-care practitioner in finding solutions for possible medical problems like sleep apnea or chronic pain. It may be worth investing in a good mattress or bed as well.

Ways to achieve more rest and better sleep include:

- Taking naps if you need to.

- Using your bedroom only for sleep and/or sex.

- Keeping all computers and electrical gadgets in a different area from where you sleep.

- Avoiding stimulating activities close to bedtime.

- Avoiding big meals within two hours of sleeping.

- Developing a meditation practice and doing a meditation prior to sleep in addition to your daily routine.

- Taking a relaxing bath in the evening.

wanting some grandchildren once or twice and raving about your sister four times. Strategically, you continue filling up her wine glass, hoping that if she gets drunk, she might excuse herself to bed early.

By the end of the night you are exhausted, and your back is stiff and sore. You lie down and fume. You run through the evening in your mind, livid at how nothing is ever good enough for your mother. You sleep fitfully.

The next morning you awaken to your alarm clock and race out of bed to shower. While leaning over to grab the soap, you suddenly feel that little twinge in your lower back again. This time, however, the twinge turns into a stabbing pain that shoots from the base of your spine up to the middle of your back, taking your breath away. You collapse to your knees, unable to move. In tears you wonder at the unfairness of your circumstance—naked in a shower, writhing in pain, too embarrassed that you will need to call your mother (of all people!) to help, and completely freaked out that something very serious is wrong.

You do the only thing you can. You crawl out of the shower, grab a towel to cover yourself, and cry, "Mom!" Your mother, of course, arrives to the rescue, as she always seems to do when it comes to you.

What just happened? You have never had back problems before!

The human body was created to move, to walk, and to run. It was not meant to be as sedentary as our human bodies are now. Rather than hunt and gather, we drive to the grocery store, order everything else online, and sit at a desk, working at a computer to earn a salary. Instead of walking over to our neighbor's, or over long distances to see relatives, we e-mail or phone home. Rather than squat to gather food, we use machinery.

When we do walk, many choose stilettos and high fashion over comfort and support. Our posture is usually bent over, because we are looking at or working on something. We exercise, but in a limited ca-

CHAPTER NINE

Stand Up for Your Spine!

I've cried, and you'd think I'd be better
for it, but the sadness just sleeps, and it
stays in my spine the rest of my life.

—CONOR OBERST, "THE CITY HAS SEX"

Your mother is coming for a visit, and your house is a mess. You are anxiously cleaning and rearranging furniture in an attempt to avoid her disapproval. Everything needs to be perfect. You pick up something heavy and feel a little twinge in your lower back. It feels a little like when a rubber band snaps. You ignore it. There is no time.

You continue working, even though your lower back aches. You ignore it, more concerned about how you will manage with your mother for two entire days. The house clean, you move on to cooking, wondering why you bother and that maybe you should have planned to a restaurant.

That evening, your mother is in rare form, only complaining

pacity, on a treadmill or at an aerobics class. When we do move, it is intermittent, and the back muscles, joints, legs, pelvis, and feet are not resilient or strong enough to bear excessive exertion or heavy lifting, especially when they are out of alignment to begin with. Throw in some emotional or stress components and a parent, sibling, or partner who triggers your feelings of inadequacy, and your back, especially your lower back, is done for.

The good news is that your spine is amenable to being strengthened, aligned, and healthy. And because your spine supports you, protects your nervous system, and enables you to stand upright, when your spine is healthy, your ability to feel supported, stay calm in the face of stress, and stand tall and self-assured can also improve, even when facing a critical parent.

Because I was in a serious car accident at the age of fifteen and then again at thirty-two, my back has taken a significant beating. I have rarely gone a day without experiencing some level of pain. At times, the pain has even brought me to my knees, leaving me immobilized for hours. After being immobilized one too many times, I decided to have a talk with my back.

I closed my eyes, concentrated on the area of pain, and asked my back why the pain was still there. My back actually answered by showing me my pattern. Every time I lost trust, when I started worrying about my future, my life, about being a failure or not being perfect, about being alone and having no one to rely on but myself, my back would "give out." The pain would not start immediately, but would gradually increase, as I persisted in ignoring my needs, devaluing myself and my life, and neglecting my self-care habits, because I was too impatient to get something done or to succeed.

The message I received from my back was that I had to learn to trust and to be patient—to trust that I was supported and valued and to be patient because I could trust that everything would turn out okay. By trusting, I could slow down, take time to take better care of myself, and allow my life to unfold as it needed to. As patience was never my strong suit, this advice seemed right on. And over the years, as I learned to cultivate more patience and trust, the exacerbations became less frequent, less severe, and shorter lasting. When I took up CrossFit and strengthened my core physically, so that I could now trust my body, the pain became minimal and fleeting, occurring only when I engaged in a strenuous physical activity. Now I pay attention to the little warning signs and take care of the problem before it becomes debilitating. I have also fortified my strength, stability, and trust in feeling supported and cared for, not just through physical fitness, but also through developing a strong community, loving relationships, and a more resilient and self-loving state of mind.

You want to build up the spine's functions—to help you stand upright, feel stable and supported, be flexible in your movement, and maintain your balance—in all aspects of your life. What should you expect from this chapter? You know the drill by now. Plan to:

- Press the PAUSE button and become acquainted with the anatomy and functions of the spine.

- OPTIMIZE your awareness of how the spine supports you along with the nervous system, what can go wrong, the signs and symptoms to watch out for that tell you to get medical help, and what you can learn from wisdom traditions and their view of the spine.

- Discover how your spine speaks to you about its positioning or your life, as you WITNESS your physiology through guided exercises.

- EXAMINE underlying emotions or beliefs that may be weakening your ability to stand tall, feel secure, or be balanced.

• Develop the tools that help you RELEASE negative habits and beliefs that are taxing your spine, RELIEVE your spine of stress and
the causes of misalignment, and RESTORE power to your back.

PAUSE and OPTIMIZE Your Awareness of Your Spine

Anatomy and Functions

Your spine is made up of twenty-four vertebral bones. Your neck, or
cervix, has seven vertebrae; your mid-back, or thoracic spine, has
twelve; and your lower back, or lumbar spine, has five. If the bones were
fused to one another, you would have one very stiff and sturdy spine,
but it would lack mobility and flexibility. To allow for more movement
and suppleness, you do have a cushion, or intervertebral disc, lying in
between each of the vertebrae.

The disc is only a cushion; it does not attach the vertebrae to each
other. You also need to have some kind of access to nutrients, some sort
of electrical setup, and a place for all the nerves going to and from the
brain. In other words, you need other surrounding structures to help
with stability, support, and ultimately movement.

Connecting one vertebra to the next is a bone structure called the
lamina, which also surrounds the nerves running down the spine,
forming the spinal canal. Each lamina has a spinous process, or a piece
of bone that juts out of the back, which you can feel if you run your
hand down your spine. Jutting out of each side of the lamina are two
more bones, called the transverse processes. Muscles attach here. Finally, what ultimately allows for more stability are the two facet joints
pointing upward and the two pointing downward that enable the vertebrae to be interlocked with one another.

If you only had a spine that was connected to two legs, you still would not have much mobility, flexibility, or balance. The spine, therefore, rests on the sacrum, a big bone wedged between your hips. The sacrum stabilizes the hips, so that you can stand upright and move forward on two legs. At the very end of the spine you have what is thought to be a remnant of a tail, also known as the coccyx. It is unclear what the purpose of the coccyx is, but because it is attached to so many muscles and ligaments, if it is out of alignment or dislocated, it can be a big source of lower-back pain.

You are able to move and maintain a sense of proprioception, or balance, largely because of the bundles of nerves between the vertebrae that run back and forth between the brain and the muscles, skin, and bones. And because of this intercommunication, one part affects the others. If the bones are weak, inflamed, or injured, the muscles will take over by tightening in an effort to preserve your stability and support. If your pelvis is tilted from sitting in a strange position for hours on end, the muscles will contract, having gotten the message that it is best for you to stay in this position. If a disc is bulging, it can compress a nearby structure, like a nerve root, which can lead to feelings of numbness, weakness, or pain in the part of the body that the nerve supplies, all of which becomes worse when you are under stress because the muscles are more contracted.

Causes and Risk Factors

There are many causes for back pain, though most of the time they are mechanical, including muscle spasms, tense muscles, sprains, fractures, and ruptured or degenerated discs. In the acute setting, back pain usually occurs, because arthritis is acting up or you have sustained some kind of injury from an activity or accident that has put stress on the bones, muscles, and tissues. Individuals more prone to succumbing to back problems have the following characteristics, histories, or behaviors:

- Are over thirty years old.

- Are less physically fit.

- Are overweight.

- Eat a diet high in calories and fat, both of which increase weight gain and inflammation.

- Have a history of arthritis.

- Have a job that requires a lot of heavy labor.

- Have diseases in other internal organs, such as kidney stones, a kidney infection, blood clots, or bone loss.[3]

The Spiny Facts

- According to the Global Burden of Disease in 2010, lower-back pain was the leading cause of disability worldwide and is the fifth most common reason for visiting an internist.[1]

- More than 26 million Americans between the ages of twenty and sixty-four experience frequent back pain.[2]

- According to these statistics, chances are that you already have experienced some back problems or that you will in the future.

Put some of these factors together in any combination—a sedentary lifestyle, heavy lifting, infection, a fall, inflammation, and emotional stress—and you might also find yourself leaning over to get some soap, only to experience stabbing back pain that brings you to your knees. Studies show, for example, that chronic interpersonal stress is associated with greater production of inflammatory cytokines.[4] The more the stress response is activated, the more the muscles tense, pulling the spine farther out of alignment and provoking further pain, pain exacerbated by an unhealthy diet that causes more inflammation and extra weight on the spine.

Red Flags That Tell You to Seek Medical Attention

Most people with back pain can usually improve within three months, using anti-inflammatory medication, massage, spinal manipulative therapy, muscle relaxants, physical therapy, and the like. However, there are certain signs and symptoms that indicate you should seek immediate medical attention.

- Steroid use or osteoporosis, which increase the possibility of bone fracture

- A major trauma to the body and a possible fracture

- A history of cancer, which, if recurring, may have spread to the spine

- Unexplained weight loss, which can point to a more serious problem like infection or cancer

- A persistent fever or a history of poor immune function, which may suggest infection

- Incontinence, or severe or progressive nerve deficits

You want to act responsibly when it comes to your spine and these red flags, as it is not worth risking the possible outcome of paralysis or even death. Don't wait until the last minute to see your doctor to find a cure or to alleviate persistent symptoms. Your goal is to pay attention to any issues you already have with standing upright, moving fluidly, being flexible, and feeling supported or balanced.

Spine Wisdom of Ancient Traditions

Thousands of years ago, MRIs and X-ray machines did not exist. Humans did not have direct access to the brain or the spine or a thorough understanding of neurons. According to wisdom traditions, the spine, especially the bones that comprise the spine, represents your strength, the very essence that allows you to stand upright, stay balanced, walk, run, get food, build shelter, and ultimately *survive*. These bones are supported by muscles and ligaments, which give you flexibility, agility, and bouncing power. The bones are also aligned in a straight line, the bottom part pointing toward the earth, the top toward the heavens.

To the ancients, the spine of a human being mirrored the tree standing tall in nature. In order for the tree to stand tall, they believed, the roots need to dig deep into the earth. It needs the support to push upward. It also needs open space to spread its branches, grow its flowers, and reach its full potential. With roots firmly in the earth and an open stance, a tree will remain stable and more flexible, despite strong gusts of wind. If not rooted firmly in the earth, it will be at the mercy of any passing storm.

This is true too in human life. When we are firmly grounded or rooted within a community or family, when we feel our finances are adequate or plentiful, and when our body is healthy, strong, and being nurtured with the right foods and exercise, we are more likely to stand tall and move through life with confidence. If we do not believe the "soil will hold" or that we are supported or safe, if our body feels weak, we have less strength and motivation to grow, thrive, and make our dreams a reality.

I think most of us can acknowledge that the fear of not being supported enough to reach our dreams or to pay our bills leads to more stress and worry, and we find ourselves often feeling as if we are bracing against the unknown. Our muscles tighten. Our nerves fire. Our sympathetic nervous system warns the rest of the body against danger, and the immune system kicks into fight-or-flight mode. If this state persists, disease, especially one that involves pain, is more likely to occur. In contrast, during those times that we feel confident or secure, when we trust that our needs will be taken care of, we are more likely to also feel relaxed, at ease, and pain-free.

Merging Science and Wisdom Traditions

Safety and security are basic human needs, and learning to trust and hope that your needs will be met by the external world in which you exist is a key component in childhood development. According to developmental psychologist Erik Erikson, trust versus mistrust is learned in the first stage of development, in the first eighteen months of life.[5] In this first period of life, you are completely dependent on your parents for food, love, warmth, and shelter, and you have to trust blindly that you will be provided for. When your needs are consistently and lovingly met, you not only develop a sense of security and attachment to your parents, but also to your environment in general. You develop the ability to trust that you can be loved and supported by the world, and that come what may, you will have what you need to survive.

Without this consistency and care, you are less likely to develop a strong sense of attachment to or trust in others, the environment, and even yourself, especially if the lack of care and love continue into the next stage of your development, when you are a toddler. It is at this stage, according to Erikson, that you learn self-confidence and self-control. You learn to walk, do things on your own, and start exploring as you are reassured and watched over by your parents, who are there to help you, should you fall or put the wrong thing in your mouth. With parental neglect, overprotection, abuse, or disapproval, you are less likely to develop confidence; instead, you acquire self-doubt and insecurity about your own abilities to handle uncertainty.

Though we may not recall it, most of us have had experiences in our early life that relate to feelings of not being secure, safe, or supported. Perhaps your parents did not support your exploration of a different path. Perhaps your family typically is not demonstrative with love and affection, meaning they rarely hug or say, "I love you." Or perhaps you grew up with love, but your family had little money and your parents were always worried. Or maybe you were born prematurely and spent the first month of your life in the hospital, away from your mom. You may or may not be consciously aware of this memory, but according to wisdom traditions, your back is.

My patient Clarisse learned for herself of some deep-seated memories that were adding to the stress that was weakening her spine. Clarisse was forty-three years old when she came to me complaining of lower-back pain, which had progressed over the past few weeks to include hip pain on both sides. She said that the pain came and went and seemed to be worse when she was sitting and better when she was walking or running. She also found stretching and crossing her legs painful. She did not have any numbness or weakness anywhere, just pain.

Upon further questioning, Clarisse did admit that she had been under a lot of stress, but this was nothing new. She always had a tendency to be overwhelmed, no matter the stress level. It was her norm, in other words, to be worried and anxious. In fact, she wondered why I was even asking, as she did not think the back or hip pain had much to do with anything emotional or psychological. She had always been anxious, and this pain was new.

Rather than going into an involved explanation of how her ongoing anxiety could be related to her pain, I instead asked Clarisse if she would be open to doing a guided exercise to further explore the pain in her back.

I began, "Bring your awareness to the base of your spine and inhale and exhale, so that the base of your spine opens and closes with your breath.

"Now imagine that the base of your spine is relaxed, open, and connected to earth. Take a few deep breaths and note how this feels.

"Now imagine that the base of your spine is tense, closed, and disconnected from the earth. Take a few deep breaths and note how this feels.

"Imagine again that the base of your spine is relaxed, open, and connected to earth. Take a few deep breaths and notice if there was a change or difference.

"Think about your current life. What is happening in your life right now? What is frustrating to you? What are you scared of?"

Then I asked Clarisse if the base of her spine felt open and relaxed or closed and tense.

"It felt open and relaxed," she said, "but when I thought about my life, it closed and it felt tenser."

I told her to imagine she was shining a flashlight at the base of her spine, right where she felt the most tension. Then I asked her whether the area was lit up or remained hidden in the dark.

"I see a small area of light, but it is mostly dark," she said.

"How far does the darkness extend?" I asked.

"It extends out to my hips."

I told her to step up close to the dark area, then imagine she could touch the area. "What does it feel like?" I asked.

"It feels like a tight muscle."

"What else do you feel? Does it have a voice?"

"It feels closed, like it is saying, 'Don't come close. Don't come in here.'"

"Can you ask it why it is there and why it doesn't want you to come close?"

"It says, 'I am bracing. I am bracing against being hurt. I do not trust that everything will be okay. I don't want to get hurt, and I don't want to be alone.'"

"Why would you get hurt? Who is going to hurt you? Why do you think you will end up alone?"

"Because I am stupid," Clarisse said.

"Why would you call yourself stupid?" I asked. "You have accomplished so much in your life."

"Because I am stupid. My dad used to call me stupid and said that it was a good thing I was pretty, because then someone would marry me. I couldn't read right away until my teachers realized I had dyslexia."

I gave Clarisse some time to cry, collect her thoughts, and let the connection between her experience and her pain settle in. When she was ready, we talked more about her fears, her beliefs, and how they were showing up in the current challenges in her life. She admitted to always feeling uncertain about her future; she never felt confident that she was smart enough or had the right skills to provide for herself. She invariably found herself in one relationship after another, because the alternative was being alone. The problem was that her boyfriends were usually abusive, at least emotionally, often putting her down or calling her "stupid," as her current boyfriend did. She was too embarrassed to tell her family or friends and often felt alone despite being in the relationship. She believed that if she worked harder, tried harder, or improved her looks, her boyfriend would be kinder and she would no longer get hurt.

As she gave words to her fears, Clarisse was able to see the discrepancy between these beliefs and the truth. The truth was that she was not stupid—she had managed to get a master's degree in teaching and was an exceptional teacher for children with learning disabilities. The truth was that she had used her own experience of hardship as a foundation to help others in the same predicament. The truth was that she was a person of value and integrity and that she indeed had a lot of love and support in her life, including her family and friends. She was not stupid and certainly not alone.

Clarisse's journey for healing her back involved working on these distorted beliefs; incorporating healing exercises that would help her reprogram new beliefs around trust, self-value, and security; connecting more deeply with her social support system; getting regular body work like massage; paying closer attention to her nutrition; and doing physical activity that was less taxing on her spine than running as well as exercises to improve her posture and flexibility. The process took about three months, and eventually Clarisse found that the pain in her hip and lower back completely subsided. She felt relaxed and at peace. She also found that she had additional courage and confidence to believe that the best possible outcome could be attainable and that it was time to try being on her own for a while.

Now it is your turn.

WITNESS the Physiology of Your Spine

AWARENESS EXERCISE

Close your eyes.

Empty your mind as you breathe in deeply and exhale completely for at least three cycles of your breath.

Bring your awareness to the base of your spine.

Inhale deeply and imagine that, as you do so, the base of your spine opens. Exhale completely and imagine that the base of your spine closes.

Get a feel for what the spine feels like when it opens and closes. Notice the contrast.

Breathe in and out slowly and, as you do so, move your awareness slowly and gently up your spine and back down, taking note of sensations.

Then ask your spine to open, and notice what you feel. Ask your spine to close, and notice what you feel.

Ask your spine to relax, and notice what you feel. Ask your spine to tense, and notice what you feel.

Ask your spine to connect itself to the heavens at the top of your head and to the earth from the base of your spine, and notice what you feel.

Ask your spine to shut off the connection at the top of your head and the base of your spine, and notice what you feel.

Now imagine you are destitute—you have little money. You do not know how you will pay your bills. You do not know if you will have enough to eat. (If this doesn't resonate for you, you can reflect on a current situation in your life that you are worried about and unsure of the outcome—what to do with your life, a job issue, whether a prospective partner will like you, feeling overwhelmed with responsibilities that no one seems to be able to do but you, and so on.)

What happens to your spine? Does it stay open or closed? What area seems most affected? The lower spine? The neck? The middle of your back? Where do you feel tension, if at all? What happens to your breath?

Now imagine you are safe. The earth is providing you with all that you need. The universe is providing you with solutions to all things. You are being showered with money. You have won the lottery. You have won a shopping spree. The partner of your dreams is standing beside you. Whatever you wish for is provided.

Notice what you feel.

You may want to spend a few minutes or more writing down your experience—what you felt, the thoughts, images, or emotions that came up. You may want to repeat the exercise with this in mind and then write about your experience.

EXAMINE Your Deeper
Emotions and Beliefs

You may have already uncovered some interesting stories, fears, or beliefs from the witnessing exercise. When examining the spine further, you can read yourself the following statements and notice the intensity of emotion that comes up for you. Rate the intensity on a scale from 0 to 10, where 0 means you feel nothing and the thought/answer is untrue, and 10 means you feel an extreme amount of fear or anger and the thought/answer rings very true.

Fear of No Support or Stability:

I often feel fearful about my future.

I do not trust that my needs will be met by another person. I can only rely on myself.

I am most fearful of losing my _____ (fill in, e.g., money, home, health, partner).

I am most fearful I will never find love or have a partner, and I will be all alone.

If something bad happens to me or _____ (fill in the fear) happens, I don't know what I would do or how I would manage.

Anger and Losing Balance, Flexibility, and Momentum:

When I get angry, I feel out of control.

I often feel frustrated that I have to do everything myself, especially if I want something done right or at all.

When people don't listen to me or respect me, I get very upset and push harder.

I really get upset with myself when I lose control.

People say that I am inflexible and rigid, especially when I am angry.

When you finish, choose the statement that elicits that most intense emotion and do the following exercise.

GOING DEEPER EXERCISE

Close your eyes, and allow yourself to feel this emotion.

Notice where you feel it in your spine.

You may not have a clear answer immediately, and whatever does come to mind may not make sense initially, so you may choose to close your eyes and focus on the area in your back that you observed had the most tension.

Ask your back the same questions, so that you can observe the image or belief that comes forward.

Write about your experience.

RELEASE, RELIEVE, and RESTORE

The good news when it comes to the spine is that you have a vast array of options available to you to help keep your spine healthy. You have the ability, for instance, to eat a healthy diet, which will decrease inflammation, maintain a healthy body weight, and keep your bones strong, thereby making you less prone to having problems. You can manage your stress levels and change your core beliefs to ones that are positive and loving. Your goals are to release and relieve stress—whether physical or emotional—in the spine and back, so that you can stand up tall with ease; to strengthen, stabilize, and improve mobility and flexibility of the spine and pelvis; and to create support and protection for your spine and for yourself in life. And of course, you want to release any fear, distrust, or anger you continue to harbor.

RELEASING FEAR AND DISTRUST MEDITATION

Close your eyes. Empty your mind as you breathe in deeply and exhale completely for three cycles of breath. Count to three as you breathe in and to five as you breathe out.

Bring your awareness to the base of your spine.

Breathe in slowly and count to three. Then breathe out slowly counting to five.

Do four breath cycles as you focus on the base of your spine

Now imagine you are releasing fear and anger as you exhale into the earth.

Even if you believe you have no fear or anger, imagine that you are releasing any negative emotion that you may not be aware of into the earth as you exhale for five cycles of breath.

When you are done, imagine that as you inhale you are absorbing the support, abundance, nurturance, and strength of the earth into the base of your spine. Absorb the earth's loving energy into the base of your spine for five cycles of breath as you inhale.

When you have completed the fifth cycle, become aware of the powerful, loving, gentle, and grounded energy in the base of your spine. Imagine you are allowing that energy to ground itself in the base of your spine.

Then breathe in and out slowly and gently and imagine this energy is lovingly massaging your spine as it moves to the top of your head.

From the crown of your head, continue to breathe in and out slowly and imagine this energy moving up to the sky, to the heavens, as if you are connecting with all the resources of the universe, so that you feel the grounded pull from the earth at the base of your spine and an uplifting pull from the universe, helping your spine align and stand tall.

Allow yourself to enjoy this feeling of support and alignment for three to five cycles of breath.

When you are ready, bring your awareness back to the base of your spine and imagine that when you breathe in, the combined energy of heaven and earth is moving up your spine to the crown of your head. When you exhale, the energy is moving down through the center of your body, back to the base of your spine.

Breathe up your spine and down the center of your body for three to five cycles of breath.

Repeat these words to yourself or out loud: "I trust there is a divine solution to all things. I am aligned with the grounded, gentle, and loving power of heaven and earth."

Then notice how you feel.

Now go back to the questions and answers you examined on fear and anger. See if the answers elicit the same emotional intensity and how true the thoughts/answers feel to you this time. Notice how you might answer the questions this time around, and perhaps you may wish to write this down.

Support and Stability

There are many different ways you can support your spine to keep it aligned, stable, and strong. The key word is "support." Even if you have preexisting problems with your spine, it does not mean you have to live in pain. Working on strengthening your body and your life at its core, so that you ultimately trust that you have the support you need, can enable you to move through your life with greater ease, energy, and ultimately joy. No pain is gain.

SITTING SUPPORT: Choose a seat with good lower-back support and preferably armrests. You may wish to support your lower back and the curve of your back by placing a pillow or rolled towel in the small of your back. Of course, you can always look for a chair combination that is ergonomically suited to you.

SHOE SUPPORT: Sometimes weak backs are a result of poor support that starts at your feet. You may wish to visit a podiatrist or orthopedist who specializes in foot problems to gauge what sort of support you may need in your shoes.

MASSAGE: You may also choose to see a physical therapist, massage therapist, or chiropractor to help you with realignment, stretching, and the relieving of muscle tension. Muscle and fascia tension, for instance, can cause your spine to be poorly aligned, and relieving this tension through deep tissue massage like Rolfing may enable the spine to align itself properly.

SOCIAL SUPPORT: Remember, a weak spine can be associated with the belief that you are not supported or cannot trust that your needs will be met. One way to counteract this belief is creating a strong social support network. Make a list of those you can turn to for what and when. This will enable you to see where you have what you need and what you might need to build up or create. For example, if you lost your home, whom could you stay with? If you need someone to pour your heart out to, who will listen? Do you feel you are part of a community you can turn to for support?

MEDICATION SUPPORT: My attitude toward medication is that it is a Band-Aid meant to stop the bleeding, so that you can get the help you need. When you are in severe pain, it is often difficult to function or get through even simple daily activities. Anti-inflammatory medications can temporarily alleviate pain and inflammation. The most commonly used medications are aspirin and nonsteroidal anti-inflammatory drugs like ibuprofen, naproxen, and the like. In high doses, all these drugs can be toxic, and you may experience unpleasant or serious side effects including heartburn, gastritis, liver disease, or allergic reactions. When choosing to take a medication, start with a small dosage first and see how you feel. Do not go over the prescribed dosage and, if you notice any side effects beginning to occur, stop the medication. Again, do not use any information given here as a replacement for seeing your health-care professional and checking to make sure you can take these medications safely.

Flexibility and Realignment

Excessive sitting, whether it is in front of a computer, in a car, or on a couch watching TV, can hurt your posture and weaken your back, making you more prone to back pain, neck pain, and many other physical problems. One way you can prevent these problems is by following steps that I adapted from mobility expert and physical therapist Kelly Starrett's advice to help your posture and create stability and strength in your spine:

- Stand up with your feet pointing straight forward, parallel to one another, directly under your hips.

- Screw your feet into the ground and squeeze your butt tightly. This will help bring the pelvis into a neutral position.

- Pull your lower ribs in so that your rib cage is now balanced over your pelvis.

- Slightly tighten your abdominal muscles (not too much), which will cause your pelvis and ribcage to get locked in place, creating tension and strength in your core.

- Set your head in a neutral position and screw your shoulders into a stable position. You do this by rolling your shoulders back as if your shoulder blades are trying to kiss, without trying to squeeze them too hard. Your chest will then move up and forward. Turn your hands back to neutral, so that your thumbs are facing forward.[6]

Balance and Ease of Movement

MOVEMENT AND STRETCHING: You can strengthen your back and create more flexibility through certain stretching exercises with or without incorporating the breath exercise. The goal is for you to learn to experience movement in a way that is connected to the earth. Here is an example of a stretch that will help you feel more balanced and at ease:

STRETCHING EXERCISE

Lie on your back with your arms spread out to the sides and your legs straight ahead. Allow yourself to connect to the strength of the earth; breathe in and out, and appreciate your connection with the earth.

Inhale and connect with the energy of the earth.

Exhale, as you bend your right leg at the knee (while keeping your left leg straight) and pull it toward your chest. The earth's energy is moving into your body. Practice three cycles of breath, releasing the tension as you inhale and pulling the knee toward you as you exhale.

Inhale and connect with the energy of the earth.

Exhale, raise your right leg toward the sky (at a 90-degree angle if you can). (You can use your hands, a rope, a band, or belt for support to help you keep the leg up if necessary.) As you exhale, allow the energy of the earth to move through your body. Release and pull for three cycles of breath.

Inhale and connect with the energy of the earth.

Exhale, and let your leg fall to the right side, as far out as it can go, allowing the earth's energy to move through your body. Hold this stretch for three cycles of breath.

Inhale and connect with the energy of the earth.

Exhale, and raise your right leg and let it fall to the left side, as far out as it can go, allowing the earth's energy to move through your body. Hold this stretch for three cycles of breath.

Inhale and exhale and bring your right leg back to resting position.

Perform the same sequence with your left leg.

When you are ready, stand up slowly, concentrating on feeling the connection between your feet and the earth.

Upon rising, stretch your arms toward the sky as you inhale.

Then drop your arms to your sides as you exhale.

Notice how good you feel.

EXERCISE: Exercise is essential for maintaining healthy bones. If you do have a history of osteoporosis, a herniated disc, or vertebral fracture, always check with your health-care provider for appropriate modifications of any exercise. In general, regular low-impact aerobic activities help improve endurance and strength of the spine and adjoining muscles. Weight-bearing exercises that involve moving against gravity (as discussed in the previous chapter) are also important for your spine health. You can always engage in more gentle exercises that incorporate light-impact weight-bearing movements like tai chi, yoga, or walking—especially walking outside and connecting to the earth or nature's wonders. Barefoot is best, as it allows you to truly be grounded to the earth and feel its support beneath you. By being outside and soaking in some sunlight, you will also get the benefit of more vitamin D.

STURDY SPINE NUTRITION: To maintain their strength, stability, and flexibility, you want the bones of your spine to be strong and dense, muscles and cartilage strong and relaxed, and your body weight healthy. And since a large component of pain and degeneration is due to bone loss or inflammation, you want to choose foods rich in vitamins and minerals that can help your bones stay strong and your body remain free of inflammation. For instance, calcium helps you maintain the integrity of your bones, while vitamin D, vitamin K, and magnesium assist you in absorbing and using the calcium efficiently and enabling the muscles to stay strong and relaxed.

Without going into too much detail, let's look at the different food groups and how they can help your bones:

> Vegetables and dark leafy greens can provide you with iron, calcium, magnesium, protein, and antioxidants like vitamin C. Indeed, contrary to popular belief, dark leafy greens are often a better source of calcium than dairy, which can cause an inflammatory reaction in many people.

> As you have learned, foods rich in omega-3 oils help with lowering inflammation while improving flexibility.

> Protein derived from beef, poultry, fish, legumes, eggs, and some grains benefit your collagen matrix as well as your muscles.

> Nuts and seeds can provide you with protein, antioxidants, essential fatty acids, and minerals like magnesium.

> Finally, you can acquire minerals and vitamins from whole grains like brown rice, barley, millet, and quinoa.

SUPPLEMENTS: Though not intended to replace a healthy diet, some supplements can help you reach your dietary goals. Remember, though, supplements are just that—*supplements*—not substitutes for good nutrition. Always check with your doctor regarding interaction with any medications you might be on or if you have other contraindications, like if you are pregnant, for instance. I mention supplements, because there has been some good research pointing to their benefits.

Research suggests that if you have low levels of calcium, magnesium, and vitamin D, you may lose bone mass faster and be more prone to weak bones that fracture.

> Calcium: Women should get approximately 1200 milligrams
> a day from all sources, including diet, while men should not
> exceed 600 milligrams a day.[7] For this reason, I usually recom-
> mend that only women take a supplement as recommended by
> their doctor if they are at risk for or have osteoporosis or os-
> teopenia or are postmenopausal. Otherwise, I find that making
> sure your diet is filled with calcium-rich foods is sufficient. If
> necessary, you can take 500 milligrams in the evening, as this
> can also help with good sleep.

> Vitamin D: Studies show that vitamin D can help you absorb
> calcium more efficiently.[8] Vitamin D, however, is not so readily
> available in your diet, though you can get it from fatty fish like
> salmon, beef liver, and egg yolks. Of course you can get this
> nutrient by spending some time in the sunlight, though you
> should check with your doctor if you are at risk for skin cancer.
> I do recommend that individuals living in colder climates take
> a supplement, especially since it is unclear how much vitamin D
> you are actually absorbing. It is always good to have your levels
> checked by your doctor. The recommended daily amount calls
> for 800–1000 IU a day in a supplement, and I usually have my
> patients double that dosage in the winter months or if they do
> not venture out into the sunlight.[9]

Magnesium: A study of women with osteoporosis in Israel reported significantly increased bone mineral density with a magnesium supplement of 250 milligrams a day when compared to a control group who did not take the supplement.[10] Another study showed that magnesium supplementation improves the body's synthesis of vitamin D and the structural strength of the bones.[11]

Note: There are different kinds of calcium and vitamin D supplements, although there is not much evidence to show that one is better than another. However, calcium carbonate and vitamin D are better taken with food, whereas calcium citrate is better absorbed on an empty stomach.

You may also wish to supplement with natural anti-inflammatories such as omega-3 fish oils (1000 milligrams per day) and turmeric (see package for directions). A recent study showed that supplementation with 1000 milligrams of omega-3 fish oil along with aerobic exercise was associated with a 19 percent increase in bone mineral density in postmenopausal women. The study also showed a decrease in inflammatory markers.[12]

Turmeric, an herb commonly found in curry powders, has been shown to be a potent anti-inflammatory, and a recent study found it may also protect against osteoporosis.[13] I enjoy adding turmeric to my grilled vegetables or a teaspoon to my scrambled eggs in the morning. It is also a wonderful addition to any stew or soup. Human studies still have to follow, but the research is promising.

Now sit up straight!

CHAPTER TEN

The Brain

Mind, Mood, and Memory

Everything we do, every thought we've ever had,
is produced by the human brain. But exactly
how it operates remains one of the biggest
unsolved mysteries, and it seems the more we
probe its secrets, the more surprises we find.

—NEIL DEGRASSE TYSON

The human brain is truly magnificent. Billions of brain cells influence and regulate your mood, thoughts, cognition, and every one of your bodily functions. They activate behaviors and actions that range from breathing to choosing a romantic partner. Many of your brain cells have a dynamic ability to continuously adapt and respond to new stimuli, so that the brain can reset itself and take new shape, enabling you to think, innovate, anticipate, and be a perpetually learning human being. The brain's ability to reorganize itself and form new neural connections is called neuroplasticity, a process that occurs throughout your life, which means you always have the ability to grow wiser, smarter, and happier.

As the command center of your body, the brain has varied and diverse functions. Without the appropriate care, however, these functions are compromised; instead of growing new neural connections, the brain cells you have can die. Every function of your brain requires energy and support, which come in the form of healthy nutrition, adequate fluid circulation, solid metabolic and structural integrity, and a waste-removal system that helps get rid of toxic substances. It might be hard to fathom that when you do not take care of yourself, you are also not taking care of your brain, which means you could increase your chances of, quite literally, losing your mind. But just think about how much work the brain has to do to keep you alive and active and, therefore, how much backing it must need.

The brain processes information coming in from the sensory cells on your tongue called taste buds. It distinguishes between more than ten thousand different smells coming from your nostrils. It takes in and processes nerve signals that were converted from vibrations received from the tiny bones in your middle ear, which originated from sound waves entering your ears. The brain processes these signals and determines what you are hearing and whether you like it. Your fingers, tongue, lips, and skin "feel" pressure, touch, temperature change, and pain, sending the information to the brain. The brain also tells you what you are seeing as information travels in through the cornea and iris of the eye to the retina, where light is transformed into nerve signals. You can see that a light is green, but you won't know that it means you can cross the street unless your brain does the processing and signaling that it is supposed to.

Have you ever wondered about how your brain manages to hold your memories and integrate the experiences with new knowledge, so that it could be put into practical use? What is the mechanism that allows you to automatically pick up your umbrella when you see it is raining outside and avoid the I-55 highway on your way to work because it tends to flood? You certainly didn't know what to do or how to drive, let alone how to walk, when you were born. Throughout your lifetime, your senses bring new information in to be processed, integrated with old, and stored in your memory to be used later. The more you stay active learning, processing, and having new experiences, the healthier your brain stays, as existing neural connections strengthen and new ones form.

The brain allows you to coordinate all incoming information and knowledge to be able to stand upright, move, and coordinate your actions throughout your life. Your left brain enables the right side of your body to move, and the right brain, your left side. Your brain controls both your voluntary muscle movement and involuntary muscle movement, like the muscles of your gut, lungs, and heart. It makes sure you breathe while you are sleeping and maintains your balance as you stand on one leg to kick a ball.

Your brain cannot survive without its supporting structures, which include a variety of proteins and hormones as well as bones, membranes, and fluids, all of which help the brain maintain its properties and viability. The bones of your scalp, for example, create a hard shell that protects the brain against trauma. Cerebral spinal fluid keeps the area clean and free of toxins. Special brain cells act to support and nourish the neurons that have active roles in maintaining your life.

Now that you are already engaged in thinking about how the brain works and how its functions might also relate to your own views and your life, you are ready to:

- Press the PAUSE button and become acquainted with the brain's anatomy and functions.

- OPTIMIZE your awareness of what can go wrong with the brain, the signs and symptoms to watch out for that tell you to get medical help, and how wisdom traditions address the brain and brain health.

- Discover how your brain may be speaking to you as you WITNESS your physiology through guided exercises.

- EXAMINE your emotions and beliefs, so that you can set the stage for healing, which you will do with the brain as well.

- Develop the tools that will help you RELEASE negative habits and beliefs that are taxing you, RELIEVE stress and worries, and RESTORE your brain health.

PAUSE and OPTIMIZE Your Awareness of Your Brain

Anatomy and Functions

The brain is comprised of three sections, the forebrain, midbrain, and hindbrain, which are intricately connected through a complex wiring system that enables communication, integration, processing, memory, coordination, and so forth to happen.

The spinal cord connects and conveys information between the brain and the rest of the body. Nerve impulses travel up and down the spinal cord relaying sensory input to the brain and motor instruction to the other parts of the body from the brain to stimulate voluntary and involuntary actions. There are billions of cells and electrical wires making up the nervous system and the main player is the nerve cell, or the neuron.

Neurons have a "body" and two extensions—one that carries signals to its body, called a dendrite, and one that carries signals out of its body, called an axon. For a nerve impulse to happen, electrical signals need to travel from one neuron to the next by traversing through the gap that separates them, or the synapse. It's pretty interesting, if you think about it. Like a magnet that draws metal to it, an impulse can only happen if the electrical charge in the nearby neuron attracts it. To make this happen, neurotransmitters like serotonin or dopamine are released to cause the electrical charge to change, so that the impulse is drawn to travel in a certain direction. Like a light switch that turns on and off, some neurotransmitters stimulate an impulse to move forward, while others function to inhibit the impulse from going any farther. Some neurons function to pick up sensory signals (like sound, touch, or feel) and are called sensory neurons. Others provoke or inhibit movement and are called motor neurons. Interneurons transmit the information between the sensory and the motor neurons.

The forebrain comprises your "higher brain," which gives you the means to function in a very complex world, and its structures include the cerebrum, cerebral cortex, thalamus, and hypothalamus. The cerebrum enables you to think, receive information, plan and imagine, manage executive functioning, solve complex problems, make decisions and judgments, and perform higher cognitive reasoning. It allows you to recognize words and create meaningful speech as well as translate and interpret sensory impulses like sound, taste, and sight. It controls your movement, or motor functions, and helps you hold on to your memories as you form new ones. Your cerebrum is responsible for putting all of your life experiences, memories, and thoughts together to form your personality and the intelligence and traits that are unique to you.

While the left side of the cerebrum enables you to be more detail oriented and logical, the right side is more responsible for your artistic tendencies and your ability to think abstractly. The cerebrum is made up of four lobes, which are responsible for different functions:

Frontal lobe: problem solving, reasoning, and logic

Parietal lobe: integrating sensory information, motor function, and spatial orientation

Temporal lobe: hearing and speech

Occipital lobe: vision

The outermost layer of the forebrain is called the cerebral cortex. Because the cerebral cortex is gray, it is also known as "gray matter." It is about 2 to 4 millimeters thick, has many folds (called gyrae; sing., gyrus), and six layers, each with a different composition of nerve cells and capillaries. The key roles of the cerebral cortex are to facilitate thought, consciousness, awareness, perception, language, attention, and memory. In fact, the majority of your information processing occurs here. The more folds, the better the processing.

The thalamus is an olive-shaped structure whose major role is to be a relay station for nerve impulses traveling to and from the brain stem, spinal cord, and the rest of the brain. All your sensory input, save your sense of smell, passes through the thalamus, which directs this information to the appropriate places in the cerebral cortex. You can think of the thalamus as Grand Central Station.

The hypothalamus lies below the thalamus (thus "hypo") and plays a vital role in regulating many of your bodily functions and emotions. It produces and regulates hormones and monitors the status and levels of the various hormones in your body, your level of hydration, satiety, body temperature, and feelings of safety. In other words, the hypothalamus is intricately involved in the regulation of your stress response, working as intermediary between the nervous and endocrine systems.

Finally, the limbic system includes a group of structures made up of the amygdala, hippocampus, cingulate gyrus, and mammillary bodies that are involved with your emotions and memory. It is part of the forebrain.

The midbrain and the hindbrain make up the brain stem. The midbrain is involved in motor functioning (ability to move) and is associated with your visual and auditory responses. This includes your ability to move your eyes, hear, respond to light, or dilate your pupils, functions that you need to maintain your balance and coordination.

The hindbrain extends from the spinal cord and joins the midbrain in the brain stem. It contains such structures as the pons, medulla oblongata, and the cerebellum. Collectively, these structures coordinate sleep patterns, posture, and your ability to maintain your equilibrium. The pons and cerebellum are mainly responsible for enabling coordination of complex movement. The pons acts like a message station between different parts of the brain, transmitting messages from the cortex and the cerebellum. It regulates your breathing, or rather your ability to transition from inspiration to exhalation, and also plays a role in generating your dreams. The medulla oblongata controls autonomic functions like breathing, digestion, blood pressure, and heart rate. It also functions in helping transfer messages from the brain to the spinal cord.

Several layers of tissue protect the brain, including the skin of your scalp and the bone, or skull, underneath it. Three layers of meninges separate the brain from the skull, providing protection, blood supply to the brain, and space for the cerebrospinal fluid to flow, which functions to carry beneficial nutrients in and toxic substances out of the brain.

Within the matrix of the brain, protective cells called glial cells provide support and metabolic functions for the brain, and they help with repair and maintenance. Glial cells are like parents who cook, clean, protect, and provide shelter for their young. Neurons depend on glial cells to provide them with needed energy, neurotransmitter regulation, and glutathione production, which can prevent oxidative stress. When glial cells are inflamed, they are useless, just like an incapacitated parent, which is why they need shelter and care too. For this reason, the endothelial cells that line the brain's small blood vessels or capillaries fit together very tightly to prevent toxins, foreign substances, or hormones from entering the brain. Normally, endothelial cells that line capillaries in the rest of the body have a space between them to allow substances through. The tight-fitting endothelial cells of the brain's capillaries make up the blood–brain barrier.

Since the brain is literally functioning all of the time and is quite vulnerable, with only a hard shell surrounding it (as opposed to fascia and muscles like the rest of your body), it is susceptible to a whole host of problems—ranging from head trauma; tumors or growths, such as aneurysms (thinning and out-pocketing of blood vessels); headaches; convulsive disorders; infection; stroke or cerebrovascular disease; and developmental disorders.[1]

Losing the Mind: Causes and Risk Factors

Because of the prevalence of cognitive decline as well as mental illness, the likelihood is that you know someone who has dementia or is showing early signs of it or someone who has a mental illness. In fact, it is not unlikely that you have experienced depression or anxiety yourself. I know I have, and I know that any condition involving the mind can be frightening and disconcerting. The good news is that often problems can be prevented or treated, and modern science is making headway in understanding diseases of the mind better.

Having said that, despite all the advances in science, we still have much to learn about why cognitive decline occurs. We know it can be part of the aging process and that cerebrovascular disease and other types of vascular disorders are just some causes or instigators of cognitive decline and brain degeneration. We also know that brain degeneration can negatively affect complex functions like processing, integrating information, and memory as well as simpler functions like basic communication, speech, or even walking.

Alzheimer's disease involves the deterioration of memory and mental functioning; often early signs go unnoticed, as most people dismiss symptoms as part of the aging process. Over time, as deterioration progresses, memory and judgment are lost, along with the ability to perform daily functions or maintain a sense of balance and coordination.

Mental Illness Facts

- Alzheimer's disease is the most common cause of dementia; it is estimated that more than 5 million Americans suffer from it.[2]

- Worldwide, Alzheimer's affects 35.6 million people, and there are 7.7 million new cases every year.[3]

- One in four adults suffers from a mental illness in any given year, and about half of the U.S. population will develop a mental illness sometime in their lives.[4]

Cognitive decline with aging does not affect everyone equally, though some form of it seems to occur in all aging people.[5] With aging, neurons may shrink or die, and the number of functional synapses can decline.[6] Data suggest that deterioration with age may lead to loss of brain volume, of the binding and signaling of neurotransmitters, of metabolic functioning, and of the thickness of the cortex.[7]

The rate and severity of decline with aging is influenced by:

Oxidative stress and free-radical damage

Changes or low levels of hormones

Chronic inflammation

Vascular disease

Poor nutrition and lifestyle habits

Excess body weight

Poor social network

Other medical conditions[8]

Oxidative stress and free-radical damage seem to be culprits in Alzheimer's as well.[9] If you want to get a clearer picture of how one problem influences another problem, which can lead to oxidative stress and subsequent brain damage, think about the consequences of having vascular disease or chronic high blood pressure:

Vascular disease leads to poor vascular flow.

Poor vascular flow causes an increase of cell death, impeded waste removal, and a buildup of toxins.

Brain integrity is lost because of the decline in the number of glial cells.

The buildup of toxins can lead to oxidative damage, further destroying neurons and other brain structures.

Vascular disease is not the only problem that can lead to increased oxidative stress and the subsequent damage. As you have learned, oxidative stress can also be increased by stress, poor dietary and lifestyle habits, and being overweight. Stress as well as anxiety and post-traumatic stress disorder have been shown to contribute to loss of brain volume and lower cognitive functioning and memory.[10] Interestingly, depression, according to many studies, can worsen cognitive function and worsening cognitive functioning may predispose individuals to depression.[11]

Mental Illness

Not only do mental-health issues affect one's ability to fully engage in life's activities, but they also negatively affect families and loved ones. Mental-health problems affect emotions, thoughts, behaviors, and often physical health. Symptoms range from feeling sad or being excessively worried, to addictive behavior, changes in eating habits, suicide attempts, an inability to concentrate or retrieve memories, a loss of interest in others or being with others, mood swings, and sleep disturbance. Usually a mental illness is diagnosed, because the symptoms interfere with the ability to perform daily functions, cope with stress or other life events, manage work or school responsibilities, or lead to continuous legal or financial problems.

Causes for mental-health problems like depression are not always entirely clear, but they appear to result from alterations in physiology, chemistry, or brain anatomy, which can be brought about by substance abuse, aging or degeneration, chemical imbalances, aftereffects of brain damage, other medical conditions, or genetic influences. The physiology or biochemistry of the brain is altered when there is a problem with the levels of one or more circulating neurotransmitters like serotonin, dopamine, or acetylcholine. The result is a problem with nerve conduction and the relaying of impulses. Imagine, for example, that there is something wrong with the electrical wiring in your house and the light in your room intermittently turns on and off without rhyme or reason. Though this is a very simplified example of a much more complex process, perhaps you get the picture of how disturbing alterations are to brain function and mood.

The major risk factors for developing mental illness include:

Having a biological relative such as a sibling or parent who also suffers from the condition

A history of stressful conditions or experiences in the womb, for example, if the mother incurred a severe amount of stress, consumed drugs or alcohol, or was exposed to viruses or toxins during pregnancy

A history of situational stress, such as financial distress or loss from death or divorce

A history of substance use or abuse

A history of brain trauma or damage

A history or influence of other medical conditions (due to the disease itself or the medications used to treat it)[12]

Since mental-health conditions can be so debilitating, it is a good idea to seek help sooner rather than later. You may choose to work with a therapist or counselor and, in some cases, you may need medication therapy to stabilize your biochemistry.

Whether it is mental illness, cognitive decline, a head injury, infection, or other brain problems, you should always seek medical attention if the symptoms occur suddenly. Listed below are some warning signs that you should seek help right away.

Red Flags That Tell You to Get Help

Conditions affecting the brain can be mild to severe. Unless there is evidence of acute trauma though—like a stroke, fall or injury, or loss of consciousness—most conditions can often be addressed and remedied as symptoms present themselves over time. There are some "Red Flags" to know about, however, to ensure that you seek medical help right away.

- Sudden onset of difficulty with memory, concentration, speech, or logical thought

- Unusual inability to function at work or school, especially in performing familiar tasks

- Unusual and exaggerated beliefs about the self or others that appear magical, grandiose, or paranoid, along with peculiar behavior

- High fever, neck stiffness, and an inability to look at the light

- Sudden onset of tremor, poor coordination, or loss of balance

- Complaints of having the "worst headache of my life"

- Headache, coupled with vomiting and confusion

- Paralysis of any kind, or weakness in arms or legs

- Drowsiness, confusion, or loss of consciousness after head injury

- Seizures or convulsions

- Inability to wake from sleep

- Headache that gets worse or does not go away

- Dilation of one or both pupils of the eyes

- Slurred speech

- Increased confusion, restlessness, or agitation[13]

What Wisdom Traditions Say About the Mind

Wisdom traditions often refer to the area of the body where the brain lies as a focal point for intuition, knowledge, insight, higher learning, thinking, connecting to spiritual beliefs, and alignment with the universe. In the Vedic tradition, the sixth and seventh chakras are associated with brain function and activity.

The sixth chakra, or "third eye," is located in the center of the forehead or brow and is responsible for physical, intuitive, and psychic sight. It is associated with the ability to self-reflect, see the "whole" picture, and ultimately be enlightened. It governs the eyes, face, brain, nervous system, and lymphatic and endocrine systems and thus controls the functioning of the rest of the body. It assimilates information received from the eyes, ears, nose, mouth, and skin and then transmits appropriate messages via hormones, nerves, immune cells, neurotransmitters, and "energy channels" to other parts of the body, so that you can function in your everyday life, from brushing your teeth to maneuvering your car in traffic.

When in balance, we think and see clearly, are able to view an entire picture, avoid rigid patterns of thinking or behaving, learn and apply new knowledge, and adapt to life's changes with ease. When out of balance, because appropriate messages are not sent out to the body, we become confused and live in disharmony. Symptoms can include hormonal imbalance as seen in menopause or thyroid disorders, headaches, learning difficulties, sinus or nasal problems, mental disturbance, and a propensity to develop brain tumors. Other symptoms may include dizziness, poor coordination, loss of sense perception (hearing, sight, smell, taste, or touch), excessive worry, depression, phobias, paranoia, and hypercritical thinking.

The crown chakra, which is located at the top of the skull, is associated with universal identity and our connection to the universe, the Divine, or something much larger than ourselves. It relates to pure awareness, consciousness, the ability to develop wisdom, spiritual connection, and a sense of peace. This chakra governs the brain stem, part of the spinal cord, pain centers, and nerves that control our ability to function and interact with the world. When balanced, we experience a sense of hope and positive expectation and have the ability to remove ourselves from stress and fear, as we connect to the larger picture and are able to embrace it. When out of balance, we may experience problems with trust, have an inability to see the larger pattern of life, and be unable to use intellect or rational analysis. Symptoms may include blindness, loss of coordination, deafness, a loss of nerve sensation or paralysis, and other diseases of the spinal cord, brain stem, and nervous system as well as of the endocrine (hormone) system.

Combining Science and Wisdom Traditions

Imbalances associated with the brain and the nervous system negatively affect your ability to think clearly, be fully connected to your senses, maintain your balance, stand tall in the world, maintain a positive perspective and expectation, problem-solve, adapt to life's stressors, and feel that you are not alone in the world. Both modern science and wisdom traditions agree that all the functions of the brain are intrinsic to your health and well-being in every facet of your life.

Think about how the brain functions. It senses, communicates, and transmits into action; integrates, stores, and analyzes; remembers, balances, and coordinates; and protects and supports itself by providing nourishment and waste removal.

If you are not connected to your senses, how well can you then understand and integrate what is happening around you?

If your balance is off, how does that feel or show up in your life?

When you are highly stressed, how good are you at adapting to life's circumstances, moving, maintaining perspective, or balancing yourself and your life?

How balanced are you when accessing your memory when you are charged with negative emotions? Do you remember the good, the bad, the ugly? Can you really remember clearly and utilize the information effectively?

If you are not eating nutritious foods, how can your mind or brain function at its optimal best?

When your thoughts, actions, or food intake are toxic, how well can your mind or brain clear them?

Wisdom traditions and modern science concur: when you nurture and find balance within yourself, you find balance in your mind and in your life.

Andrew complained of a long history of allergies, headaches, sinus infections, and now worsening anxiety. He was allergic to dust, pollen, dog and cat hair, and many other environmental substances. He was often nervous about traveling or going places, worried that his allergies would be set off. He also reported that he had never been able to smell anything. Andrew had been taking medications for allergies almost his entire life, and he wanted to stop.

Acupuncture had already helped tremendously, as his headaches were less frequent and his symptoms were less severe. His acupuncturist had also instructed him to take omega-3 fish oils and B vitamins and avoid dairy and refined sugar, which seemed to have helped as well.

However, he still complained that his head often felt heavy, he had pains in his head in between his eyes, and he sometimes felt dizzy. He complained of feeling a pulsating sensation in his head, which made him increasingly more anxious. A recent eye exam showed nothing abnormal. He had been so worried about his frequent headaches that he'd asked his doctor to order the appropriate tests to rule out anything life-threatening like a brain tumor.

When I asked Andrew why he thought he might have a brain tumor, he admitted that he was a "hypochondriac." He told me he worried about everything, especially his health, and he also fretted about work, a lot, especially about being fired. I asked if he had done something wrong at work, but he replied that no, he had done nothing that would merit his being fired, but he worried about it anyway. He had a hard time falling asleep, as he spent hours worrying about the details of what needed to get done the next day or because he ran scenarios through his mind over and over again, whether related to work, health, or something else.

Though it was clear that Andrew was a "worrier," it was also evident to me that he was a man who was in touch with his intuition, since he had already mentioned to me that his intuition had led him to seek holistic health treatment. This meant to me that Andrew was capable of insight, deeper thinking, and an ability to integrate the insight and act upon it. His problem was that because he was so good at it, he defaulted to overthinking to combat his fear, to give him a sense of control. Because of his fear, Andrew ended up thinking too much and not trusting his own insights or actions, preventing him from seeing and understanding situations clearly, especially those that concerned his health or his work.

With Andrew, it was important to help him feel a sense of trust, to lower stress-response reactivity, and to provide him with coping tools that could replace his need to overthink. One of the strategies was showing him how to connect with the support of heaven and earth, just as you learned to do in the spine chapter. He learned to use his breath to empty his mind and induce a deeper sense of relaxation. This exercise alone helped Andrew experience feelings of peace and, more important, quiet.

I asked Andrew to practice this imagery and breath exercise a minimum of twice a day, perhaps every morning and every evening. He was also to use it anytime he felt his worries were overshadowing his ability to think or see clearly. I encouraged him to continue acupuncture and the dietary and supplement recommendations. Over the next few visits, Andrew's headaches stopped, his allergies further improved, and he found that he worried less. He was even able to laugh at himself for some of the things that had troubled him.

Now it is your turn.

WITNESS the Physiology of Your Brain

As you have learned thus far, witnessing involves not so much a visualization of structures, but of sensations you experience in particular areas of the body. This time, you will be scanning the entire head—this includes what you might feel behind your eyes, behind your forehead, or at the base of your skull. Notice where you may feel tension, ache, or even a sense of light-headedness.

AWARENESS EXERCISE

Breathe in slowly for three counts. Breathe out slowly for five counts.

Do this several times as you empty your mind, allowing thoughts to flow out into the wind.

Scan every area of your head, the top of your head, your forehead, in between your eyebrows, behind your eyes, your sinuses,

your ears, the center of your head, the area in front of the back of
your skull, the base of your skull, and so on. Each time you get to a
new area, say to yourself, "I am worried," and notice what you feel
and experience.

Make sure you take your time with each area, using your breath
count of three in and five out.

Now scan each of the areas again, this time saying to yourself,
"There is a divine solution to all things," and see what happens.

You may wish to write about your observations when you are ready
or simply keep in mind where you felt the most discomfort or tension.
Then prepare yourself to dig deeper and see what lies beneath.

EXAMINE Your Deeper Emotions and Beliefs

Read through these statements and choose one or more that ring most
true, which you can gauge by the strong response or feeling that a statement elicits. Write down the ones that feel the most true for you.

Trust and Hope Versus Stress and Fear:

Life has shown me that I cannot trust that I will have what I
need in the future, and I have to work hard to make sure I do. I
have to think about everything now.

There is no higher power, God, or universal Spirit. We are alone
in this world.

I am scared of dying or of getting sick.

I am afraid of ending up alone.

Communication and Speech:

I can't seem to communicate clearly, especially when I am angry or upset.

I worry that I won't be heard or understood.

I worry I won't understand others.

If I speak up, I will get hurt.

Intuition and Insights:

I can't trust my own feelings, because I seem to always make the wrong choice.

It's safer to seek the advice of others.

I am not sure if what I am sensing is real, or if I am just an anxious person.

Wisdom and Integration of Knowledge:

I can't make meaning of some of the difficult situations I have been through.

I am really angry, critical, anxious, upset, or fearful because of what happened to me.

If someone hurts me, you bet I will get my revenge.

Balance and Coordination:

I can't seem to get my balance. Every time I think I am going to, something bad happens to me.

I am easily upset or angered.

I have a hard time doing more than one thing at one time.

I am really uncoordinated.

Symptoms:

> I often get headaches or dizziness.

> I often have trouble sleeping, either falling asleep or staying asleep.

> I have frequent sinus problems.

> I often have problems with my vision, hearing, taste, or smell that are worsening.

Once you have chosen the statement(s), do the following:

GOING DEEPER EXERCISE

Close your eyes and bring your awareness back to the area of your head where you experienced discomfort in the witnessing exercise and allow yourself to think about one of the statements.

Take note of the sensations you experience and also the subsequent thoughts that arise to support the statement.

Take five or more minutes to write down what you felt or experienced and then why you feel this statement is true and what the evidence is to support it. Try not to think too hard and write freely, letting all the emotions and beliefs come forward. You can do this for as many statements as you wish, but usually two or three are sufficient to elicit the predominant negative story that is supporting the thoughts.

RELEASE, RELIEVE, and RESTORE

As was true for Andrew, one of your primary goals is to work on releasing distrust and fear to enable your brain to function at its optimal best. By doing so, you help your brain because you are lowering stress-response reactivity and therefore ridding your brain of toxins, improving its oxygenation, decreasing oxidative stress, enabling access to higher brain functioning so that you can think more clearly and make wiser decisions, and stimulating the natural process of growth and plasticity of your neurons.

Opening the Senses and the Gateway of Communication

With a closed mind, you cannot see the big picture or what is around you. When the stress response is overactive, your ability to connect with higher thinking and reasoning is shut off. Your tendency will be to feel victimized or hurt easily by life's circumstances, so that life will seem more like a struggle. You can instead learn to open your mind and allow yourself to feel more expansive and connected to your own and the world's resources using your senses. When you do so, you open the gateway of communication with your higher self, your body, and with others. You also learn to see all situations in life as opportunities for growth and learning, rather than hardships yet to come.

OPENING THE MIND MEDITATION

Begin your slow, deep breathing, breathing in for three counts, and breathing out for five.

For four cycles of breath, empty the mind.

You are emptying your thoughts, giving them to the earth, to Mother Earth.

Mother Earth will transform your thoughts for you, just like she brings life after a forest fire. Relax into Mother Earth.

For four cycles of breath, empty the tension in the entire spine. Release everything to Mother Earth. Relax into Mother Earth.

For four cycles of breath, empty any tension in your shoulders, arms, hands, legs, and feet as you release everything to Mother Earth. Relax into Mother Earth.

For four cycles of breath, empty any tension in your heart, lungs, and abdomen. Release everything to Mother Earth. Relax into Mother Earth.

For four cycles of breath, completely let go and relax into Mother Earth. Like a seed that has been planted in her soil, allow yourself to receive support and nurturance. You imagine you are being given the support and energy to grow through the earth, through the world, to expand toward the stars. Your mind opens, your heart blooms like a flower, and possibilities expand all around you.

For four cycles of breath, the sun shines down into your mind, down your spine, and into the earth, creating a line made of light connecting you to heaven and earth, helping you stand upright and balanced.

For four cycles of breath, observe the healing light, as it moves up your spine and down through your center. Repeat these words as often as you wish, "I am connected to all things, to all beings, and to the wisdom of the universe."

Once you have completed this exercise, review what you wrote during the examination portion. You may notice that the intensity you previously experienced when you read specific statements is either gone or reduced. Reflect on how the words you wrote down may not seem so true now, and perhaps write down the evidence that shows the contrary. In other words, if you felt that you could never trust your own feelings, try to find instances when you trusted your feelings or hunches and they ended up being right.

COMMUNICATION IN ACTION: Any activity that involves a repetitive practice causes the brain to transmit signals in a specific pattern over and over again, allowing for connections between neurons to strengthen, so that eventually the task at hand is easier and easier to accomplish. For this reason, regular exercise or performance of a physically difficult task becomes more fluid over time. The ability to lift weights, however, does not really help you build neuronal connections for getting better at playing golf. You would have to practice that too. Interestingly, if you practice a given mental task repetitively, neuronal connections and synapses in other pathways do get stronger. For instance, getting better at playing chess can help you get better at driving a car.[14] Similarly, if you played golf and engaged your higher thinking and cognition while playing the sport, this would positively affect your cognition in other areas.

PRACTICING DEEP LISTENING: Communication involves both giving and receiving of information, and to get by in our world this means with other people. Whether you have a brain injury or you simply are stressed, communication can be challenging when you have problems listening and integrating information, speaking your needs or truth clearly, and being aware of social cues or other people's nonverbal ways of communicating. Especially when your negative emotions get the best of you and you have less access to your higher brain functioning, you might find yourself selectively listening and saying (or not saying) things you regret later.

A wonderful practice to get used to is the art of deep listening and speaking. The "deep" happens when you allow yourself to take a pause, a deep breath, that provides you with the space and time you need to fully hear words and take in the surrounding nuances as well as speak from a heartfelt place rather than a stressed one. The tenets of this practice, as I teach my patients, are:

Decide to not be in a rush to speak or listen. Allow yourself to wait, take a pause, to ensure all the information is coming in and being processed.

Breathe. Inhale deeply and exhale completely, so that you can bring the mind and body system into a place that is more calm and receptive.

Listen and speak with your heart. Work on emptying your mind and bring your awareness to your heart when you listen or speak. Try to engage all of your senses.

Write first. If you feel emotionally charged about something, practice a witnessing exercise or write out your thoughts first to see if you can gain some clarity within yourself and your emotions.

Create a safe place to rant. Sometimes you just need to rant, to get whatever is on your mind out without holding back, and writing doesn't cut it. Choose a friend, therapist, or counselor whom you know you can safely speak to without worrying that you might be judged for what is going on inside you. Let the person know that you do not need advice, but you need an outlet to express your negative emotions fully, because they are really blocking you from communicating well with others.

Memory, Knowledge, and Integration

CREATIVE ACTIVITY: The plasticity of your brain can be maintained throughout your life through physical activity and continued mental and cognitive stimulation. Studies show that even individuals who display clinical cognitive impairment can see significant improvement in functioning when they undergo cognitive training exercises in which intellectual capacity is challenged.[15] One study revealed that intensive cognitive training for eight weeks improved blood flow to the prefrontal cortex versus no change in blood flow in the group that was exposed only to educational material without the cognitive training.[16]

Cognitive training includes a myriad of activities for your mind and can be learning something new, like a new language or how to play chess. These two activities are well known to improve cognitive functioning. There are also many things you can do easily right now. You can try writing with your opposite hand, learn a new direction to drive to work, type or scroll with the opposite hand, combine your senses by engaging in mindfulness when eating (smelling and tasting), or eating while listening to music with your eyes closed. You can also read more, see if you can recall what you have read and write it down, write your own creative story, watch less TV, and play more board games—from word games like Scrabble or Boggle to bingo and dominos—which stimulate your thinking as well as hand–eye coordination. And remember to have fun! The more fun you have, the more your neurons have room to grow and reshape themselves.

SLEEP ON IT: You can probably recall several times when you were sleep deprived and unable to remember where you put your keys or what you went into the kitchen to get. You cannot operate in your best capacity when you are sleep deprived. Your problem-solving abilities, creativity, critical thinking skills, and life-managing capabilities all suffer. Even more so, as studies show, you need sleep for learning, memory, and synaptic plasticity.[17] How do you know you are getting enough sleep? You feel rested when you wake up in the morning, not after you've had your first cup of coffee (see Chapter 4 for sleep recommendations).

HAVING FUN WITH FRIENDS: Social support will help you feel safe and, in addition, less alone. We know that loving friendships and relationships help us get through hardships, and indeed social support helps with depression and anxiety symptoms. Interestingly, new research is revealing that such support may also provide protection against strokes by reducing the amount of inflammation that can damage the brain.[18] Remember the love hormone, oxytocin? Studies have shown that it is partially responsible for enabling you to focus on your table mate in a loud restaurant. Oxytocin seems to enable your brain to quiet background activity while enhancing the accuracy of impulses being stimulated to fire, so that the activity of brain circuits is essentially sharpened. The study, built upon research done in Geneva thirty years ago, showed that oxytocin worked on the hippocampus, the part of your brain involved in memory and cognition.[19]

And really, these findings are not surprising. Is an infant more likely to focus on your face or begin to walk or talk in a noisy and stressful environment or in one that is nurturing and loving? Having loving and supportive relationships boosts not only your emotional health, but also your brain health. Throw in fun and laughter, and multiple regions of the brain are now engaged to be vital and active.

Balance and Coordination

STRESS REDUCTION AND RELAXATION PRACTICES: As I mentioned previously, stress and its aftereffects are a major cause of brain dysfunction or of at least making any existing problem worse. Every time you engage in an activity or lifestyle habit that decreases the reactivity of your stress response, you are strengthening your brain and enhancing your higher brain function. I strongly recommend starting a meditation practice of your choosing, perhaps ten to twenty minutes a day. This can include, of course, mindfulness practices, which can help with improving your brain function as you integrate the use of different senses. Science does show that meditation can have lasting positive effects on brain function. In one study it was found that the more years a person had been meditating, the more gyrification was revealed on an MRI. Gyrification refers to the folding of the cerebral cortex.[20] The more of it you have, the better your brain is at information processing.

Other stress-reduction techniques can involve cognitive restructuring exercises, laughter or humor therapy, exercise, working with a counselor or therapist, practicing breath-focusing exercises throughout the day, or engaging in a spiritual practice or ritual like prayer.

SPIRITUALITY AND CONNECTING TO SOMETHING LARGER: If you are not up to joining a spiritual community, there are other ways for you to engage in activities that enable you to connect to something larger than yourself. Oxytocin can be released through hugs and affection, but similar effects can occur through altruistic action, spiritual or religious activities, meditation or prayer, and being out in nature. Aside from the meditation practice you experienced in this chapter, being out in nature is one of the easiest ways to accomplish this task. Whether the cause is a reduction in inflammation and stress hormones or an increase of oxytocin or stimulation of brain reward centers, studies show that spending time out in nature is good for you and your brain. You want to especially think about getting outside to get your vitamin D, as this vitamin has been found to be important for brain health as well. Studies at UCLA have found that vitamin D along with curcumin may help stimulate the immune system, so that it clears plaque in the brain due to Alzheimer's.[21] Fifteen minutes a day of sun without sunscreen on your arms and legs a few times a week should do the trick.

Self-Protection and Support

GETTING PHYSICAL: Every time you perform a mental or a physical task, the massive neural network in your brain is stimulated. When you engage in a wide range of activities that require engagement of different muscle groups, the plasticity, or ability to grow and change, of your synapses and neurons is positively influenced. Studies show that physical exercise enhances cognitive function, and one reason may be because it increases levels of brain-derived neurotrophic factor (BDNF), a protein that improves learning, memory, and higher thinking by stimulating growth of new neurons, helping existing neurons stay alive, and helping the functioning of synapses.[22]

A recent comprehensive analysis of fifteen studies looking at 33,000 subjects followed for twelve years found that those who had the highest amount of physical activity were 38 percent less likely to show signs of cognitive decline.[23] Even better, physical activity also improves mood, while decreasing stress, as endorphin levels rise and cortisol levels fall. A Harvard Medical School study in 2005 found that walking fast for thirty-five minutes a day five times a week significantly (positively) influenced mild to moderate depression.[24]

What does this mean? Move your body. Do different things to engage a variety of muscle groups. If you do not use it, you lose it. Walk outdoors where the terrain is not so predictable, so that you are perfecting your balance. Practice yoga or tai chi to practice flow of movement, engagement of muscles, and balance. Get your heart rate up to the appropriate level for you for fifteen minutes a few times a week. Have fun! If you don't, you won't go back for more.

FOOD TO BOOST THE BRAIN: What you eat, why you eat, and how you eat directly affect your brain structure and function. Have you ever noticed when you eat a lot of junk food, including bread, sugar, or fried foods, you feel fuzzy, somewhat sick, and tired? If you are like me, you may have noticed that you feel irritable, fatigued, depressed, or anxious the next day.

When thinking about nutrition for your brain, recall that its metabolic rate is quite high, so it requires nutritious foods that can be efficiently used for fuel. Diets high in fat and simple sugars are harmful to the brain, inducing an inflammatory cycle, poor insulin regulation, and oxidative stress. Multiple studies have found a correlation between such poor food choices and cognitive functioning or worsening mood disturbances.[25]

It appears that with these dietary habits, brain cells can become resistant to insulin, so that they are eventually unable to obtain the glucose they need to function and live. Glucose levels remain unused, causing blood-sugar levels to stay high. High blood-sugar levels are toxic to your neurons, as the excess sugar binds to protein molecules to make advanced glycolytic enzymes (AGEs), which in turn enhance oxidative stress and free-radical damage.[26] The end result is that you have brain tissue damage along with poor energy intake by the brain cells.

In contrast, the Mediterranean diet provides vegetables, colorful fruits, healthy grains, and foods that are rich in good fats that support friendly gut bacteria. Studies show this diet improves insulin sensitivity, fat breakdown, metabolism, depression, and life span.[27] Such healthy eating benefits the brain, as it reduces inflammation and oxidative stress and also provides healthy fats needed for cells and membranes. A study of 1,393 people who were followed over four and a half years showed that those individuals who adhered best to the Mediterranean diet had a 28 percent lower risk of developing cognitive impairment than those who had poor adherence.[28]

What does this mean for you and your brain?

The Mediterranean diet is high in *omega-3 fish oils,* which are essential for a healthy brain, both for its structure and its functions, including neurotransmitter signaling and production. Fish like salmon, trout, herring, sardines, kippers, and mackerel are good sources of omega-3. Other good sources include flaxseed oil, pumpkin seeds, walnuts, hazelnuts, sesame seeds, sunflower seeds, and cashews.

New research is also showing that *coconut oil* may be helpful in preventing or treating neurodegenerative diseases. One small study of 152 patients with Alzheimer's disease showed that cognitive scores improved within forty-five to ninety days after supplementation with coconut oil.[29] You can put a tablespoon in your coffee or tea in the morning or use coconut milk instead of regular milk to enjoy the benefits. Of course, any fat that improves circulation and cardiovascular help is good for your brain health. This includes the monounsaturated fat you get from avocados.

Since the brain is highly susceptible to oxidative stress, enhancing the natural *antioxidants* in your body can help your brain stay healthy. Multiple studies have pointed to the benefit, for instance, of blueberries on memory, learning, and overall cognitive performance.[30] Though most research has been done in animals, new studies looking at memory and cognitive function in humans point to the benefits of an antioxidant called pterostilbene, found to significantly improve cognitive functioning and memory.[31] Other antioxidant-rich foods that help keep free radicals in check include other berries; fruits and vegetables like carrots, spinach, and red grapes; drinks like green tea, red wine, and coffee; and dark chocolate (in moderation, of course).

A plethora of studies have been pointing to the benefits of the *B vitamins* for brain health. Vitamin B1 or thiamine, for example, may help regulate blood-sugar levels, while B12 and folic acid are needed for better cognitive functioning and nervous-system health. Many legumes provide a rich dietary source of B-complex vitamins, while meat, poultry, and fish are excellent B12 sources. A study done at the University of Oxford found that supplementation with folic acid, vitamin B6, and vitamin B12 for two years lowered levels of homocysteine and the amount of brain shrinkage in individuals diagnosed with mild cognitive impairment.[32] Homocysteine is an amino acid that may be linked to Alzheimer's disease.

PHYSICAL SUPPORT: If you plan on really taking care of yourself, you want to take care of your head. Feeling and being secure in your life enable you to be more at ease, think more clearly, and maintain a more open attitude and flexible nature when dealing with obstacles or stress. This sense of security not only comes from the social support you can build around you, but also physical support. In other words, wear a helmet when riding a bike, scooter, motorcycle, skateboard, snowboard, or horse or when playing aggressive contact sports like hockey, football, or baseball, where there is a chance of being hit in the head by a hard ball. Wear your seatbelt in all motor vehicles. Improve lighting in your home, and make sure carpeting is installed correctly so that you avoid tripping. And work on your physical strength and ability to maintain your balance with such exercises as yoga, tai chi, or other forms of martial arts.

When your brain is not functioning at its best, you cannot be you and you can't fully take care of the rest of your body. Even if you only follow some of the suggestions in this chapter, you will find that you have managed to change your health destiny for the better.

The New Strong You, in Your Power, Changing Your Health Destiny

I t is my sincere hope that this book has brought you closer to understanding the incredible power your mind and body have within themselves to heal, to be strong and resilient, even when challenged by life's obstacles or genetic predispositions. Perhaps now you can begin to discover what being "strong" really means—that it is not just about being able to lift heavy weights or manage problems without asking for help; it is about having and being enough to handle anything. It is a state of resilience that entails knowing you have access to a great power within yourself to heal and thrive.

When you live in a state of fear and stress you lose access to that power and you become vulnerable to disease and hardship, rather than venerable. When you own your power, you know you are venerable. Your core is strong, and your belief is that you are aligned with internal and external resources to mitigate uncertainty. Your stress response is used to generate action and is not wreaking havoc on the rest of your body. As a result, your energy is continuously regenerated and renewed, enabling you to stay vital and vibrant. Getting to this place involves not only setting up and nurturing your resources, but also trusting them to work.

Learning to live this new strong paradigm has been a personal journey for me. It has taken many years for the left-brained academic in me to relax and accept the notion that it is okay not to know everything or have all the answers, that every one of us has a myriad of resources available to us that support our natural ability to be strong and heal and that don't always include drugs or something that is scientifically validated.

I had forgotten the world I had been brought up in as a child, where my father's mother made us herbal teas when we fell ill or threw water at our car as we left her house to ward off evil or accidents and to ensure a safe trip. I had forgotten that at six years old I wanted to be like her, a strong woman, a mother, a person of faith, and a healer. I had forgotten that, at the very least, I wanted to be able to run as fast as the car.

We left my grandmother's world when I was only seven, moving from Israel to the United States, where I was now surrounded by scientists and academicians like my father. In this new world I was influenced by the interesting conversations and came to the recognition that I had to do something with my life that would bring security, esteem, and money. I went from wanting to be a medicine woman, to wanting to be the bionic woman, to wanting to be a doctor. And in the process of becoming a doctor, I forgot about the rest and focused on the science.

It would be twenty years later that I would finally set out on a journey to suspend my usual state of disbelief and delve into the world of spirituality and healing again. It would take me that long to figure out that all my dreams were valid—of being a medicine woman, a resilient being who could be rebuilt and renewed like the bionic woman, a teacher and a healer; that there was validity in the provisions of both modern medicine and ancient healing practices. That we need to be both healthy and strong became clear when my mother got sick.

March 8, 2013, witnessed one of the worst snowstorms Boston had seen in decades. It was also the day my mother dropped, unconscious, to the kitchen floor as a result of a sudden pulmonary embolism and cardiac arrest. She was resuscitated many times, and the doctors in the emergency room and later in the intensive-care unit (ICU) told us her prognosis was extremely poor. Even if she survived, she would likely have brain damage, as no one knew how long her brain had gone without oxygen.

Mom spent ten days in the ICU, being kept alive by multiple medications, blood transfusions, a ventilator, and twenty-four-hour nursing care. We never left her side. We had the hospital volunteer Reiki practitioners come in daily; we had healers and prayer circles around the globe working on and praying for Mom. Each time the medical team thought that we might lose her or that she might not survive yet another complicated procedure, she came through. More than once the medical team would stare at Mom in awe, not fully understanding how or why she continued to recover. We often heard them say she was truly a miracle, especially the day Mom's condition really turned the corner, so that she was able to be weaned off the medication and the ventilator.

I will never forget the moment she opened her eyes and smiled, as she saw her husband's face smiling back at her. She improved every day thereafter, coming home six weeks later. She healed almost completely, and no one, including the amazing medical team, knows completely how and why. The medical team told us she was a walking miracle and that her journey is a testament to incredible advances in modern medicine, the healing power of love, and healing modalities we do not understand as well as the triumph of her spirit to live on. Today, Mom is stronger than she was before the event. She takes better care of herself, exercising, eating more healthy foods, and engaging in activities that bring her joy, like painting.

As for me, the experience enabled me to become "aligned" with my abilities as a physician, meditator, and healer. I used my medical knowledge and intuition to help make decisions with the medical team. I did "energy work" on my Mom several times a day, placing my hands on her body and drawing in love and positive energy from the universe to be transmitted through me to her. When I wasn't busy being with Mom, I meditated, I ate only the healthy foods my body needed to be fueled, I slept as I could, and I cried when I needed to, letting myself be wrapped up by those I love and trust. Though I was frightened, I also knew somewhere deep within me that ultimately Mom's pulling through was up to her, or perhaps her spirit, and her own will to live. She had to want to come back. The best medical team in the world couldn't make that decision for her. Dr. James M. Kirshenbaum, the amazing cardiologist on service, said as much.

I learned to trust in the process of life and that I had resources within me and around me to handle pretty much anything. And with this trust, with this deep inner knowing that I had all that I needed to mitigate uncertainty, I became strong, mentally, emotionally, and physically.

You see, trust is a state of being, much like helplessness or hopefulness. It is a willing state of vulnerability and surrender based on the expectation that your own, another person's, or the universe's, God's, nature's, or a "higher power's" intentions and actions are altruistic, beneficial, and skillful enough to ensure a positive outcome. In other words, trust represents the inner knowing that you can expect good even when life throws curveballs. It means you trust your body, and your body trusts itself. This knowing allows you to access a state of inner peace, whereby your stress response is quieted, your mind is clear, and your body is relaxed.

When you are in a constant state of stress, whether you are worried about something or continuously poisoning your body with processed foods, this trust, this inner peace is not possible. When this goes on for too long, power is lost, and distrust or fear takes over. The body's natural ability to heal is hindered.

The good news, as you have learned, is that you can always change from one state to another. You now have the tools to do so. Each and every one of us has the ability to change our health destiny. We all have access to the same resources, to the same POWER.

It is our choice whether we use them.

Acknowledgments

This book would not have come into fruition were it not for my agent, Scott Hoffman, and Gideon Weil and Claudia Boutote from HarperOne, who realized my voice still needed to be heard. I thank the entire HarperOne team for their incredible support, diligence, and enthusiasm. In that light, I thank Amy Parsons for introducing me to Claudia Boutote and therefore the entire HarperOne family.

Special thanks to my wonderful family—Jacob, Shirley, Julie, Eliya, and Maia Selhub—for their love and support. I am so grateful to have both my parents with me to celebrate this book and their own victories over illness.

It is with the love, laughter, and support from my "soul family"—my CrossFit community and friends, especially my soul-sisters Venita Bell Shaw, Kimberly Wallace, Chiara Piovella, Lisa Ross, Sharon Freedman, Michelle Pinage, Beth Hamacher, Karen von-Kleist Dobos, Rebecca Lovejoy, Faith Murphy, Linda Sacks, Celeste Yacobini, Felicity Broennan, and Stasia Forsythe Siena—that I found my voice and the courage to bring forth my knowledge and ideas in this book, so it is with deep gratitude that I thank you all.

Lastly, I thank my clients and patients who continue to teach me and grace me with the opportunity to participate in their journey to changing their health destiny.

Notes

Chapter 1: The Power to Transform Health

1. H. N. Rasmussen, M. F. Scheier, and J. B. Greenhouse, "Optimism and Physical Health: A Meta-Analytic Review," *Annals of Behavioral Medicine* 37/3 (June 2009): 239–56.

2. Sara Rimer, "Happiness and Health," *Harvard School of Public Health News,* Winter 2011, http://www.hsph.harvard.edu/news/magazine/happiness-stress -heart-disease/.

3. R. Orozco-Solis, and P. Sassone-Corsi, "Epigenetic Control and Circadian Clock: Linking Metabolism to Neuronal Responses," *Journal of Neuroscience* 264 (April 4, 2014): 76–87; doi: 10.1016/j.neuroscience.2014.01.043.

4. D. Landgraf, A. Shostak, and H. Oster, "Clock Genes and Sleep," *Pflügers Archiv* 463/1 (January 2012): 3–14; doi: 10.1007/s00424-011-1003-9.

5. Manoj K. Bhasin et al., "Relaxation Response Induces Temporal Transcriptome Changes in Energy Metabolism, Insulin Secretion and Inflammatory Pathways," *PLoS One* (May 1, 2013); doi: 10.1371/journal. pone.0062817.

6. J. K. Zubieta and C. S. Stohler, "Neurobiological Mechanisms of Placebo Responses," *Annals of the New York Academy of Sciences* 1156 (March 2009): 198–210; doi: 10.1111/j.1749-6632.2009.04424.x.

7. Walter Cannon, *The Wisdom of the Body* (New York: Norton, 1932); *Bodily Changes in Pain, Hunger, Fear, and Rage* (New York: Appleton-Century-Crofts, 1929).

8. Hans Selye, "Stress and Disease," *Science* 122 (October 1955): 625–31.

9. Bruce McEwen, *The End of Stress as We Know It* (New York: Dana, 2002).

Chapter 2: Choosing Healthy, Choosing Happy

1. Emeran A. Mayer and Kirsten Tillisch, "The Brain-Gut Axis in Abdominal Pain Syndromes," *Annual Review of Medicine* 62 (2011): 381–96; doi: 10.1146/annurev-med-012309-103958.

2. Michael Gershon, *The Second Brain: A Groundbreaking New Understanding of Nervous Disorders of the Stomach and Intestine* (New York: Harper Perennial, 1999).

3. P. N. Tobler et al., "Reward Value Coding Distinct from Risk Attitude-Related Uncertainty Coding in Human Reward Systems," *Journal of Neurophysiology* 97/2 (2007): 1621–32.

4. David Burns, *Feeling Good: The New Mood Therapy* (New York: New American Library, 1980).

5. S. S. Luthar, D. Cicchetti, and B. Beck, "The Construct of Resilience: A Critical Evaluation and Guidelines for Future Work," *Child Development* 71/3 (2000): 543–62.

6. T. Baumgartner et al., "Oxytocin Shapes the Neural Circuitry of Trust and Trust Adaptation in Humans," *Neuron* 58/4 (May 2008): 639–50.

7. T. Baumgartner, *BBC News*, May 21, 2008.

Chapter 3: POWER Your Way to Health

1. Eckhart Tolle, *The Power of Now* (Novato, CA: New World Library, 1999).

2. S. Praissman, "Mindfulness-Based Stress Reduction: A Literature Review and Clinician's Guide," *Journal of Academic Nursing Practitioners* 20/4 (April 2008): 212–16.

3. R. J. Davidson et al., "Alterations in Brain and Immune Function Produced by Mindfulness Meditation," *Psychosomatic Medicine* 65/4 (July–August 2003): 564–70.

4. Z. Fadel et al., "Mindfulness Meditation Improves Cognition: Evidence of Brief Mental Training," *Consciousness and Cognition* 19/2 (June 2010): 597–605.

5. Ted Kaptchuk, *The Web That Has No Weaver: Understanding Chinese Medicine*, 2nd ed. (Chicago: Contemporary, 2000).

6. Deepak Chopra, "Chakras," http://www.chopra.com/community/online-library/terms/chakras.

7. M. R. Irwin et al., "Sleep Deprivation and Activation of Morning Levels of Cellular and Genomic Markers of Inflammation," *Archives of Internal Medicine* 166/16 (September 2006): 1756–62.

8. A. L. Berg et al., "The Effects of Adrenocorticotrophic Hormone and Cortisol on Homo-cysteine and Vitamin B Concentrations," *Clinical Chemistry and Laboratory Medicine* 44 (2006): 628–31.

9. David A. Camfield et al., "The Effects of Multivitamin Supplementation on Diurnal Cortisol Secretion and Perceived Stress," *Nutrients* 5 (2013): 4429–50; doi:10.3390/nu5114429.

10. A. L. Pizent et al., "Serum Copper, Zinc and Selenium Levels with Regard to Psychological Stress in Men," *Journal of Trace Elements in Medicine and Biology* 13/1–2 (July 1999): 34–39.

11. L. Mascutelli, F. Pezzetta, and J. L. Sullivan, "Inhibition of Iron Absorption by Coffee and the Reduced Risk of Type 2 Diabetes Mellitus," *Archives of Internal Medicine* 167/2 (January 2007): 204–5.

12. D. E. R. Warburton, C. W. Nicol, and S. S. D. Bredin, "Health Benefits of Physical Activity: The Evidence," *Canadian Medical Association Journal* 174/6 (March 2006): 801–9.

13. Warburton, et al., "Health Benefits of Physical Activity," 801–9.

14. G. S. Passos et al., "Is Exercise an Alternative Treatment for Chronic Insomnia?" *Clinics* 67/6 (June 2012): 653–59.

15. B. N. Uchino, "Social Support and Health: A Review of Physiological Processes Potentially Underlying Links to Disease Outcomes," *Journal of Behavioral Medicine* 29/4 (August 2006): 377–87.

16. J. Levin, "How Faith Heals: A Theoretical Model," *Explore (NY)* 5/2 (March–April 2009): 77–96.

17. Herbert Benson and Miriam Z. Klipper, *The Relaxation Response* (New York: Harper-Torch, 2000).

18. G. B. Stefano and T. Esch, "Love and Stress," *Neuroendocrinology Letters* 26/3 (June 2005): 173–74.

19. G. D. Jacobs, "The Physiology of Mind-Body Interactions: The Stress Response and the Relaxation Response," *Journal of Alternative and Complementary Medicine* 7, Suppl. 1 (2001): S83–92.

20. Manoj K. Bhasin et al., "Relaxation Response Induces Temporal Transcriptome Changes in Energy Metabolism, Insulin Secretion and Inflammatory Pathways," *PloS One* 8/5 (May 1, 2013): e62817; doi:10.1371/journal.pone.0062817.

Chapter 4: The Immune System: Your 24-Hour Security System

1. Cancer Research UK Press Release, "Cancer Is the Biggest Fear, but 34 Percent Put It Down to Fate," December, 2010, http://info.cancerresearchuk.org/news/archive/pressrelease/2010-12-08-cancer-is-biggest-fear-but-some-think-it-is-fate.

2. Christopher Jacob, "Top 5 Killer Cancers," *Health Guidance,* http://www.healthguidance.org/entry/15796/1/Top-5-Killer-Cancers.html.

3. K. Chong-Hang, "Dietary Lipophilic Antioxidants: Implications and Significance in the Aging Process," *Reviews in Food Science and Nutrition* 50/10 (November 2010): 931–37.

4. Chart of the immune system: http://www.virtualmedicalcentre.com/uploads/VMC/Anatomy/Immune_system_large.jpg.

5. American Cancer Society, "Cancer Facts and Figures," 2002, http://www.uhmsi.com/docs/CancerFacts&Figures2002.pdf.

6. M. A. Dooley and S. L. Hogan, "Environmental Epidemiology and Risk Factors for Autoimmune Disease," *Current Opinion in Rheumatology* 15/2 (March 2003): 99–103; "Link Between Common Lifestyle Factors, Immune System and Cancer," *Medical News,* November 13, 2006, http://www.news-medical.net/news/2006/11/13/20965.aspx.

7. "Annual Report to the Nation on the Status of Cancer, 1975–2009, Featuring the Burden and Trends in Human Papillomavirus (HPV)–Associated Cancers and HPV Vaccination Coverage Levels," *Journal of the National Cancer Institute,* February 5, 2013, http://jnci.oxfordjournals.org/content/early/2013/01/03/jnci.djs491.full.

8. American Cancer Society, "Cancer Facts and Figures," 2002, http://www.uhmsi.com/docs/CancerFacts&Figures2002.pdf.

9. American Cancer Society, "Cancer Facts and Figures."

10. Mahima et al., "Immunomodulators in Day to Day Life: A Review," *Pakistan Journal of Biological Sciences* 16/17 (September 2013): 826–43.

11. M. F. Holick and T. C. Chen, "Vitamin D Deficiency: A Worldwide Problem with Health Consequences," *American Journal of Clinical Nutrition* 87/4 (April 2008): 1080S–6S; K. Yin and D. K. Agrawal, "Vitamin D and Inflammatory Diseases," *Journal of Inflammation Research* 7 (May 2014): 69–87.

12. S. F. Bloomfield et al., "Too Clean, or Not Too Clean: The Hygiene Hypothesis and Home Hygiene," *Clinical and Experimental Allergy* 36/4 (April 2006): 402–25.

13. "Immune Deficiency," http://www.jaxallergy.com/immune-deficiency.php.

14. "CDC Fast Facts A-Z," Vital Health Statistics, 2003.

15. "Chronic Conditions: A Challenge for the 21st Century," National Academy on an Aging Society, 2000.

16. "Autoimmune Statistics," American Autoimmune Related Disease Association, 2004, https://www.aarda.org/autoimmune_statistics.php.

17. "Autoimmune Statistics," American Autoimmune Related Disease Association.

18. "Cancer Facts and Statistics," American Cancer Society, 2013, http://www.cancer.org/research/cancerfactsstatistics/.

19. "Cancer Facts and Statistics," American Cancer Society.

20. A. W. Tang, "A Practical Guide to Anaphylaxis," *American Family Physician* 68/7 (October 2003): 1325–33.

21. D. E. R. Warburton, C. W. Nicol, and S. S. D. Bredin, "Health Benefits of Physical Activity: The Evidence," *Canadian Medical Association Journal* 174/6 (March 2006): 801–9.

22. D. Haaland et al., "Is Regular Exercise a Friend or Foe of the Aging Immune System? A Systematic Review," *Clinical Journal of Sports Medicine* 18/6 (November 2008): 539–48.

23. S. Stea, A. Beraudi, and D. De Pasquale, "Essential Oils for Complementary Treatment of Surgical Patients: State of the Art," *Evidence Based Complementary and Alternative Medicine* 2014, ID: 726341, http://dx.doi: 10.1155/2014/726341; T. Atsumi and K. Tonosaki, "Smelling Lavender and Rosemary Increases Free-

Radical Scavenging Activity and Decreases Cortisol Level in Saliva," *Psychiatry Residence* 150/1 (February 28, 2007): 89–96; M. Komiya, T. Takeuchi, and E. Harada, "Lemon Oil Vapor Causes an Anti-Stress Effect via Modulating the 5-HT and DA Activities in Mice," *Behavioural Brain Research* 172/2 (September 25, 2006): 240–49, II. G. Preuss et al., "Effects of Essential Oils and Monolaurin on Staphylococcus Aureus: In Vitro and In Vivo Studies," *Toxicology Mechanisms and Methods* 15/4 (2005): 279–85.

24. K. Kawakami et al., "Effects of Phytoncides on Blood Pressure Under Restraint Stress in SHRSP," *Clinical and Experimental Pharmacology and Physiology* 31, Suppl. 2 (December 2004): S27–28.

25. B. J. Park, Y. Tsunetsugu, and Y. Miyazaki, "The Physiological Effects of Shinrin-yoku: Evidence from Field Experiments in 24 Forests Across Japan," *Environmental Health and Preventive Medicine* 15/1 (January 2010): 18–28.

26. V. F. Gladwell et al., "The Great Outdoors: How a Green Exercise Environment Can Benefit All," *Extreme Physiology and Medicine* 2/1 (January 2013): 3.

27. J. DeWolfe, T. M. Waliczek, and J. M. Zajicek, "The Relationship Between Levels of Greenery and Landscaping at Track and Field Sites, Anxiety, and Sports Performance of Collegiate Track and Field Athletes," *HortTechnology* 21/3 (June 2011): 329–35.

28. J. R. Davidson, H. Moldofsky, and F. A. Lue, "Growth Hormone and Cortisol Secretion in Relation to Sleep and Wakefulness," *Journal of Psychiatry and Neuroscience* 16/2 (July 1991): 96–102.

29. M. R. Irwin et al., "Sleep Deprivation and Activation of Morning Levels of Cellular and Genomic Markers of Inflammation," *Archives of Internal Medicine* 166/16 (September 2006): 1756–62.

30. K. Kour and S. Bani, "Chicoric Acid Regulates Behavioral and Biochemical Alterations Induced by Chronic Stress in Experimental Swiss Albino Mice," *Pharmacology, Biochemistry and Behavior* 99/3 (September 2011): 342–48.

31. M. Ligor, T. Trziszka, and B. Buszewski, "Study of Antioxidant Activity of Biologically Active Compounds Isolated from Green Vegetables by Coupled Analytical Techniques," *Food Analytical Methods* 6/2 (April 2013): 630–36.

32. L. Galland, "Magnesium and Immune Function: An Overview," *Magnesium* 7/5–6 (1988): 290–99.

33. Y. Xy and S. Y. Qian, "Anti-Cancer Activities of W–6 Polyunsaturated Fatty Acids." *Biomedical Journal* 37/3 (2014): 112–19.

34. C. A. Daley, A. Abbott, and S. Larson, "A Review of Fatty Acid Profiles and Antioxidant Content in Grass-Fed and Grain-Fed Beef," *Nutrition Journal* 9 (March 2010): 10; doi:10.1186/1475-2891-9-10.

35. D. G. Armstrong et al., "Effect of Oral Nutritional Supplementation on Wound Healing in Diabetic Foot Ulcers: A Prospective Randomized Controlled Trial," *Diabetic Medicine* 31/9 (September 2014): 1069–77; doi: 10.1111/dme.12509.

36. C. Ceapa et al., "Influence of Fermented Milk Products, Prebiotics and Probiotics on Microbiota Composition and Health," *Best Practice and Research Clinical Gastroenterology* 27/1 (February 2013): 139–55.

37. Debra Umberson and Jennifer Karas Montez, "Social Relationships and Health: A Flashpoint for Health Policy," *Journal of Health and Social Behavior* 51, Suppl. (2010): S54–S68.

38. S. D. Pressman et al., "Loneliness, Social Network Size, and Immune Response to Influenza Vaccine in College Freshmen," *Health Psychology* 24/3 (May 2005): 297–306.

39. S. W. Cole et al., "Social Regulation of Gene Expression in Human Leukocytes," *Genome Biology* 8/9 (2007): R189.

Chapter 5: Opening Your Heart and Reclaiming Your Health

1. Mimi Guarneri, *The Heart Speaks: A Cardiologist Reveals the Secret Language of Healing* (New York: Touchstone, 2007), Introduction.

2. Cleveland Clinic, *Heart Facts,* http://my.clevelandclinic.org/heart/heart-blood-vessels/heart-facts.aspx.

3. J. Andrew Armour, "The Little Brain on the Heart," *Cleveland Clinic Journal of Medicine* 74/1 (2007): S48–S51.

4. Institute of Medicine (US) Committee on Preventing the Global Epidemic of Cardiovascular Disease: Meeting the Challenges in Developing Countries, *Promoting Cardiovascular Health in the Developing World: A Critical Challenge to Achieve Global Health,* ed. V. Fuster and B. B. Kelly (Washington, DC: National Academies Press, 2010), http://www.ncbi. nlm.nih.gov/books/NBK45688/.

5. World Heart Federation, *Cardiovascular Disease Risk Factors,* http://www.world-heart-federation.org/cardiovascular-health/cardiovascular-disease-risk-factors/.

6. World Heart Federation, *Cardiovascular Disease Risk Factors.*

7. G. E. Vaillant, "The Neuroendocrine System and Stress, Emotions, Thoughts and Feelings," *Mens Sana Monographs* 9/1 (January–December 2011): 113–28.

8. Rollin McCraty, "The Energetic Heart Is Unfolding," *Institute of HeartMath,* http://www.heartmath.org/free-services/articles-of-the-heart/energetic-heart-is-unfolding.html.

9. S. Reichert et al., "Use of Floss/Interdental Brushes Is Associated with Lower Risk for New Cardiovascular Events Among Patients with Coronary Heart Disease," *Journal of Periodontal Research,* May 2014; doi: 10.1111/jre.12191.

10. "American Heart Association Recommendations for Physical Activity in Adults," http://www.heart.org/HEARTORG/GettingHealthy/PhysicalActivity/StartWalking/American-Heart-Association-Guidelines_UCM_307976_Article.jsp.

11. G. B. Stephano and T. Esch, "Integrative Medical Therapy: Examination of Meditation's Therapeutic and Global Medicine Outcomes via Nitric Oxide (Review)," *International Journal of Molecular Medicine* 16/4 (October 2005): 621–30.

12. National Heart, Lung, and Blood Institute and National Institutes of Health, *Keep the Beat: Heart Healthy Recipes,* NIH publication No. 03–2921, July 2003, http://img.thebody.com/hhs/2003/heart_recipes.pdf.

13. K. Ortho-Gomer, A. Rosengren, and L. Wilhelmsen, "Lack of Social Support and Incidence of Coronary Heart Disease in Middle-Aged Swedish Men," *Psychosomatic Medicine* 55/1 (1993): 37–43.

14. H. S. Lett et al., "Social Support and Coronary Heart Disease: Epidemiologic Evidence and Implications for Treatment," *Psychosomatic Medicine* 67/6 (2005): 869–78.

15. G. Alspach, "Extending the Tradition of Giving Thanks: Recognizing the Health Benefits of Gratitude," *Critical Care Nurse* 29/6 (December 2009): 12–18; doi: 10.4037/ccn2009331.

16. M. J. Poulin et al., "Giving to Others and the Association Between Stress and Mortality," *American Journal of Public Health* 103/9 (September 2013): 1649–55.

17. R. Mora-Ripoli, "The Therapeutic Value of Laughter in Medicine," *Alternative Therapies in Health and Medicine* 16/6 (November–December 2010): 56–64.

Chapter 6: The Lungs: Letting In and Letting Go

1. "Human Lung," *Wikipedia,* http://en.wikipedia.org/wiki/Human_lung.

2. American Lung Association, "Epidemiology and Statistics, " 2013, http://www.lung.org/finding-cures/our-research/epidemiology-and-statistics-rpts.html.

3. Centers for Disease Control and Prevention, "Lung Cancer Statistics," 2010, http://www.cdc.gov/cancer/lung/statistics/.

4. Centers for Disease Control and Prevention, "Lung Cancer Statistics."

5. American Lung Association, "Lung Cancer Fact Sheet," 2012, http://www.lung.org/lung-disease/lung-cancer/resources/facts-figures/lung-cancer-fact-sheet.html.

6. National Cancer Institute at the National Institutes of Health, "A Snapshot of Lung Cancer," 2013, http://www.cancer.gov/researchandfunding/snapshots/lung.

7. National Cancer Institute at the National Institutes of Health, *SEER Cancer Statistics Review,* 1973–2008.

8. American Lung Association, "Lung Cancer Fact Sheet."

9. Anne Harding, "Twelve Ways to Keep Your Lungs Strong and Healthy," *Huffington Post,* May 2011, http://www.huffingtonpost.com/2011/05/22/healthy-lungs_n_865182.html#s281458title=Dont_smoke_.

10. Ad Vingerhoets and Lauren Bylsma, "Crying as a Multifaceted Health Psychology Conceptualisation: Crying as Coping, Risk Factor, and Symptom," *European Health Psychologist* 9/4 (December 2007): 68–74.

11. B. E. Becker, "Aquatic Therapy: Scientific Foundations and Clinical Rehabilitation Applications," *Physical Medicine and Rehabilitation* 1/9 (September 2009): 859–72.

12. S. O. Shaheen et al., "The Relationship of Dietary Patterns with Adult Lung Function and COPD," *European Respiratory Journal* 36/2 (August 2010): 277–84.

13. A. F. Abdull Razis and N. M. Noor, "Cruciferous Vegetables: Dietary Phyto-chemicals for Cancer Prevention," *Asian Pacific Journal of Cancer Prevention* 14/3 (2013): 1565–70.

14. J. D. Finklea, R. U. Grossmann, and V. Tangpricha, "Vitamin D and Chronic Lung Disease: A Review of Molecular Mechanisms and Clinical Studies," *Advances in Nutrition* 2/3 (May 2011): 244–53.

15. Harri Hemilä and Pekka Louhiala, "Vitamin C May Affect Lung Infections," *Journal of the Royal Society of Medicine* 100/11 (November 2007): 495–98.

16. A. Murakami, H. Ashida, and J. Terao, "Multitargeted Cancer Prevention by Quercetin," *Cancer Letters* 269/2 (October 2008): 315–25.

Chapter 7: The Gastrointestinal System: You Eat and You Are

1. Y. H. Yau and M. N. Potenza, "Stress and Eating Behaviors," *Minerva Endocrinologica* 38/3 (September 2013): 255–67.

2. "Digestive Diseases: The Facts," *Health Guidance,* http://www .healthguidance.org/entry/6328/1/Digestive-Diseases-The-Facts.html.

3. M. G. Welch et al., "Combined Administration of Secretin and Oxytocin Inhibits Chronic Colitis and Associated Activation of Forebrain Neurons," *Neurogastroenterology and Motility* 22/6 (June 2010): 654-e202.

4. B. Nagakgaesm, B. Peleteiro, and N. Lunet, "Dietary Patterns and Colorectal Cancer: Systematic Review and Meta-analysis," *European Journal of Cancer Prevention* 21/1 (January 2012): 15–23.

5. D. S. Chan et al., "Red and Processed Meat and Colorectal Cancer Incidence: Meta-analysis of Prospective Studies," *PLoS One* 6/6 (2011): e20456.

6. V. Hassan et al., "Association Between Serum 25 (OH) Vitamin D Concentrations and Inflammatory Bowel Diseases (IBDs) Activity," *Medical Journal of Malaysia* 68/1 (2013): 34–38.

7. S. A. Bingham et al., "Dietary Fibre in Food and Protection Against Colorectal Cancer in the European Prospective Investigation into Cancer and Nutrition (EPIC): An Observational Study," *Lancet* 361/9368 (2003): 1496–501; N. Murphy et al., "Dietary Fibre Intake and Risks of Cancers of the Colon and Rectum in the European Prospective Investigation into Cancer and Nutrition (EPIC)," *PLoS One* 7/6 (June 2012): e39361.

8. U. Volta et al., "Non-celiac Gluten Sensitivity: Questions Still to Be Answered Despite Increasing Awareness," *Cellular and Molecular Immunology* 10/5 (September 2013): 383–92.

9. National Center for Complementary and Alternative Medicine, "Oral Probiotics: An Introduction," http://nccam.nih.gov/health/probiotics/ introduction.htm; California Dairy Research Foundation, "Probiotics," http:// cdrf.org/home/checkoff-investments/usprobiotics/.

10. National Center for Complementary and Alternative Medicine, "Oral Probiotics: An Introduction."

11. M. T. Bethune and C. Khosla, "Oral Enzyme Therapy for Celiac Sprue," *Methods in Enzymology* 502 (2012): 241–71; P. M. Kleveland et al., "Effect of Pancreatic Enzymes in Non-Ulcer Dyspepsia: A Pilot Study," *Scandinavian Journal of Gastroenterology* 25 (1990): 298–301; University of Michigan Health

System, "Digestive Enzymes," http://www.uofmhealth.org/health-library/hn–2840008#hn–2840008-uses; C. Ciacci et al., "Effect of Beta-glucan, Inositol and Digestive Enzymes in GI Symptoms of Patients with IBS," *European Review for Medical and Pharmacological Sciences* 15 (2011): 637–43.

12. H. P. F. Peters and W. R. De Vries, "Potential Benefits and Hazards of Physical Activity and Exercise on the Gastrointestinal Tract," *Gut* 48 (2001): 435–39.

13. M. E. Eisenberg et al., "Family Meals and Substance Use: Is There a Long-Term Protective Association?" *Journal of Adolescent Health* 43/2 (August 2008): 151–56.

14. M. G. Welch et al., "Combined Administration of Secretin and Oxytocin Inhibits Chronic Colitis and Associated Activation of Forebrain Neurons," *Neuro-gastroenterology and Motility* 22/6 (June 2010): 654-e202; A. D. de Araujo et al., "Selenoether Oxytocin Analogues Have Analgesic Properties in a Mouse Model of Chronic Abdominal Pain," *Nature Communications* 5 (2014): 3165; doi: 10.1038/ncomms4165.

Chapter 8: The Musculoskeletal System: Move It or Lose It

1. National Library of Medicine, PubMed Health, "Fibromyalgia," http://www.ncbi.nlm.nih.gov/pubmedhealth/PMH0001463/.

2. Centers for Disease Control and Prevention, "Arthritis-Related Statistics," http://www.cdc.gov/arthritis/data_statistics/arthritis_related_stats.htm.

3. P. Primatesta, E. Plana, and D. Rothenbacher, "Gout Treatment and Comorbidities: A Retrospective Cohort Study in a Large US Managed Care Population," *BMC Musculoskeletal Disorders* 12/103 (May 2011); doi: 10.1186/1471-2474-12-103.

4. "The Burden of Musculoskeletal Diseases in the United States," http://www.boneandjointburden.org/.

5. C. R. FitzSimmons and J. Wardrope, "Assessment and Care of Musculoskeletal Problems," *Emergency Medicine Journal* 22/1 (2005): 68–76.

6. P. L. Hill and N. A. Turiano, "Purpose in Life as a Predictor of Mortality Across Adulthood," *Psychological Science* (May 2014); doi: 10.1177/0956797614531799.

7. Centers for Disease Control and Prevention, "Physical Activity and Arthritis Overview," http://www.cdc.gov/arthritis/pa_overview.htm.

8. I. Hafstrom et al., "A Vegan Diet Free of Gluten Improves the Signs and Symptoms of Rheumatoid Arthritis: The Effects on Arthritis Correlate with a Reduction in Antibodies to Food Antigens," *Rheumatology* 40/10 (2001): 1175–79.

9. G. Howatson et al., "Influence of Tart Cherry Juice on Indices of Recovery Following Marathon Running," *Scandinavian Journal of Medicine and Science in Sports* 20/6 (December 2010): 843–52; K. S. Kuehl et al., "Efficacy of Tart Cherry Juice in Reducing Muscle Pain During Running: A Randomized Control Trial," *Journal of the International Society of Sports Nutrition* 7/7 (May 2010):

17; M. Cesari et al., "Antioxidants and Physical Performance in Elderly Persons: The Invecchiare in Chianti (InCHIANTI) Study," *American Journal of Clinical Nutrition* 79/2 (February 2004): 289–94.

10. P. C. Calder, "Fatty Acids and Inflammation: The Cutting Edge Between Food and Pharma," *European Journal of Pharmacology* 668/1 (September 2011): S50–S58; S. Hurst et al., "Dietary Fatty Acids and Arthritis," *Prostaglandins, Leukotrienes, and Essential Fatty Acids* 82/4–6 (April–June 2010): 315–18.

11. S. M. Robinson et al., "Diet and Its Relationship with Grip Strength in Community-Dwelling Older Men and Women: The Hertfordshire Cohort Study," *Journal of the American Geriatrics Society* 56/1 (January 2008): 84–90.

12. W. B. Grant, "The Role of Meat in the Expression of Rheumatoid Arthritis," *British Journal of Nutrition* 84/5 (November 2000): 589–95.

13. Institute of Medicine, "Dietary Reference Intakes: Water, Potassium, Sodium, Chloride, and Sulfate," February 11, 2004, http://www.iom.edu/ Reports/2004/Dietary-Reference-Intakes-Water-Potassium-Sodium-Chloride -and-Sulfate.aspx.

14. K. J. Ruff, D. P. DeVore, and M. A. Robinson, "Eggshell Membrane: A Possible New Natural Therapeutic for Joint and Connective Tissue Disorders: Results from Two Open-Label Human Clinical Studies," *Clinical Interventions in Aging* 4 (2009): 235–40.

Chapter 9: Stand Up for Your Spine!

1. D. Hoy et al., "Measuring the Global Burden of Low Back Pain," *Best Practices Research in Clinical Rheumatology* 24/2 (April 2010): 155–65.

2. National Centers for Health Statistics, *Chartbook on Trends in the Health of Americans with Special Feature on Pain,* 2006, http://www.cdc.gov/nchs/data/hus/ hus06.pdf.

3. National Institute of Arthritis and Musculoskeletal and Skin Diseases, National Institute of Health, "What Is Back Pain?" September 2009; http://www .niams.nih.gov/Health_Info/Back_Pain/back_pain_ff.asp.

4. G. E. Miller, N. Rohleder, and S. W. Cole, "Chronic Interpersonal Stress Predicts Activation of Pro- and Anti-Inflammatory Signaling Pathways 6 Months Later," *Psychosomatic Medicine* 71/1 (January 2009): 57–62.

5. Arlene F. Harder, "The Developmental Stages of Erik Erikson," http://www.support4change.com/index. php?option=com_content&view=article&id=47&Itemid=108.

6. Kelly Starrett with Glen Cordoza, *Becoming a Supple Leopard: The Ultimate Guide to Resolving Pain, Preventing Injury, and Optimizing Athletic Performance* (Riverside, NJ: Victory Belt, 2013), 29–30.

7. National Institutes of Health, "Calcium: Dietary Supplement Fact Sheet," http://ods.od.nih.gov/factsheets/Calcium-HealthProfessional/.

8. A. Felsenfeld, M. Rodriguez, and B. Levine, "New Insights in Regulation of Calcium Homeostasis," *Current Opinion in Nephrology Hypertension* 22/4 (July 2013): 371–76.

9. National Institutes of Health, "Vitamin D: Fact Sheet for Health Professionals," http://ods.od.nih.gov/factsheets/VitaminD-HealthProfessional/.

10. C. T. Price, J. R. Langford, and F. A. Liporace, "Essential Nutrients for Bone Health and a Review of Their Availability in the Average North American Diet," *Open Orthopedics Journal* 6 (2012): 143–49.

11. K. M. Ryder et al., "Magnesium Intake from Food and Supplements Is Associated with Bone Mineral Density in Healthy Older White Subjects," *Journal of the American Geriatrics Society* 53 (November 2005): 1875–80.

12. B. Tartibian et al., "Long-Term Aerobic Exercise and Omega-3 Supplementation Modulate Osteoporosis Through Inflammatory Mechanisms in Post-Menopausal Women: A Randomized, Repeated Measures Study," *Nutrition and Metabolism* (London) 8 (October 2011): 71.

13. L. E. Wright et al., "Protection of Trabecular Bone in Ovariectomized Rats by Turmeric (Curcuma longa L.) Is Dependent on Extract Composition," *Journal of Agricultural and Food Chemistry* 58/17 (2010): 9498–504.

Chapter 10: The Brain: Mind, Mood, and Memory

1. Centers for Disease Control and Prevention, "Injury Prevention and Control: Traumatic Brain Injury," http://www.cdc.gov/traumaticbraininjury/statistics.html; World Health Organization, "Headache Disorders," October 2012, http://www.who.int/mediacentre/factsheets/fs277/en/; National Institute of Neurological Disorders and Stroke, "Cerebral Aneurysms Fact Sheet," http://www.ninds.nih.gov/disorders/cerebral_aneurysm/detail_cerebral_aneurysms.htm#24173309; Mayo Clinic, "Epilepsy," http://www.mayoclinic.com/health/epilepsy/DS00342/DSECTION=risk-factors; Centers for Disease Control and Prevention, "Cerebrovascular Disease or Stroke," http://www.cdc.gov/nchs/fastats/stroke.htm; Centers for Disease Control and Prevention, "Causes and Risk Factors of Cerebral Palsy," http://www.cdc.gov/ncbddd/cp/causes.html; National Institute of Neurological Disorders and Stroke, "Meningitis and Encephalitis Fact Sheet," http://www.ninds.nih.gov/disorders/encephalitis_meningitis/detail_encephalitis_meningitis.htm; Alzheimer's Association, "Alzheimer's Disease Facts and Figures," http://www.alz.org/mglc/in_my_community_60862.asp.

2. World Health Organization, "Ten Facts on Dementia," http://www.who.int/features/factfiles/dementia/en/.

3. A. Fjell et al., "Structural Brain Changes in Aging: Courses, Causes and Cognitive Consequences. *Reviews in Neuroscience* 21/3 (2010): 182–221.

4. Mayo Clinic, "Mental Illness," http://www.mayoclinic.com/health/mental-illness/DS01104/DSECTION=risk-factor.

5. H. Horie et al., "Membrane Elasticity of Mouse Dorsal Root Ganglion Neurons Decreases with Aging," *FEBS Letters* 269/1 (August 1990): 23–25.

6. Y. Sato and T. Endo, "Alteration of Brain Glycoproteins During Aging," *Geriatrics and Gerontology International* 10, Suppl. 1 (July 2010): S32–40; E. A. Sametsky et al., "Synaptic Strength and Postsynaptically Silent Synapses Through Advanced Aging in Rat Hippocampal CA1 Pyramidal Neurons." *Neurobiology of Aging* 31/5 (May 2010): 813–25; P. Rabbitt et al., "Frontal Tests and Models for Cognitive Ageing," *European Journal of Cognitive Psychology* 13/1–2 (2001): 5–28; E. Hoekzema at al., "The Effects of Aging on Dopaminergic Neurotransmission: A MicroPET Study of [11C]-Raclopride Binding in the Aged Rodent Brain," *Neuroscience* 171/4 (December 2010): 1283–86.

7. L. Backman et al., "Linking Cognitive Aging to Alterations in Dopamine Neuro-transmitter Functioning: Recent Data and Future Avenues," *Neuroscience and Biobehavioral Reviews* 34/5 (April 2010): 670–77; C. E. Teuissen et al., "Inflammation Markers in Relation to Cognition in a Healthy Aging Population," *Journal of Neuroimmunology* 134/1–2 (January 2003): 142–50.

8. S. E. Harris et al., "A Genetic Association Analysis of Cognitive Ability and Cognitive Ageing Using 325 Markers for 109 Genes Associated with Oxidative Stress or Cognition," *BMC Genetics* 8 (July 2007): 43; O. I. Okereke et al., "Fasting Plasma Insulin, C-Peptide and Cognitive Change in Older Men Without Diabetes: Results from the Physicians' Health Study II," *Neuroepidemiology* 34/4 (2010): 200–207; J. Ryan et al., "Hormone Levels and Cognitive Function in Postmenopausal Midlife Women," *Neurobiology of Aging* 33/3 (March 2012): 617; M. A. Lovell and W. R. Markesbery, "Oxidative DNA Damage in Mild Cognitive Impairment and Late-Stage Alzheimer's Disease," *Nucleic Acids Research* 35/22 (2007): 7497–504.

9. Lovell and Markesbery, "Oxidative DNA Damage"; A. Sandstrom et al., "Cognitive Deficits in Relation to Personality Type and Hypothalamic-Pituitary-Adrenal (HPA) Axis Dysfunction in Women with Stress-Related Exhaustion," *Scandinavian Journal of Psychology* 52/1 (February 2011): 71–82.

10. J. L. Peters et al., "Interaction of Stress, Lead Burden, and Age on Cognition in Older Men: The VA Normative Aging Study," *Environmental Health Perspectives* 118/4 (April 2010): 505–10; D. W. Hedges and F. L. Woon, "Premorbid Brain Volume Estimates and Reduced Total Brain Volume in Adults Exposed to Trauma with or Without Posttraumatic Stress Disorder: A Meta-Analysis," *Cognitive and Behavioral Neurology* 23/2 (June 2010): 124–29; K. Felmingham et al., "Duration of Posttraumatic Stress Disorder Predicts Hippocampal Grey Matter Loss," *NeurorReport* 20/16 (October 2009): 1402–6; F. Panza et al., "Late-Life Depression, Mild Cognitive Impairment, and Dementia: Possible Continuum?" *American Journal of Geriatric Psychiatry* 18/2 (February 2010): 98–116.

11. E. A. Crocco et al., "How Late-Life Depression Affects Cognition: Neural Mechanisms," *Current Psychiatry Reports* 12/1 (February 2010): 34–38; M. J. van Tol et al., "Regional Brain Volume in Depression and Anxiety Disorders,"

Archive of General Psychiatry 67/10 (October 2010): 1002–11; R. C. Kessler et al., "Prevalence, Severity, and Comorbidity of Twelve-Month DSM-IV Disorders in the National Comorbidity Survey Replication (NCS-R)," *Archives of General Psychiatry* 62/6 (June 2005): 617–27.

12. Mayo Clinic, "Mental Illness."

13. M. Sobri et al., "Red Flags in Patients Presenting with Headache: Clinical Indications for Neuroimaging," *British Journal of Radiology* 76/908 (August 2003): 532–35, http://bjr.birjournals.org/content/76/908/532.full. Family Practice Notebook, "Head Injury and CT Indications in Adults," http://www.fpnotebook.com/neuro/Rad/HdInjryCtIndctnsInAdlts.htm; National Institute of Neurological Disorders and Stroke, "NINDS Traumatic Brain Injury Information Page," http://www.ninds.nih.gov/disorders/tbi/tbi.htm; MedicineNet, "Brain Damage: Symptoms, Causes, Treatments," http://www.medicinenet.com/brain_damage_symptoms_causes_treatment/article.htm.

14. M. Bedard and B. Weaver, "Cognitive Training for Older Drivers Can Reduce the Frequency of Involvement in Motor Vehicle Collisions," *Evidence Based Mental Health* 14/2 (May 2011): 52.

15. E. M. Zelinski et al., "Improvement in Memory with Plasticity-Based Adaptive Cognitive Training: Results of the 3-Month Follow-up," *Journal of the American Geriatrics Society* 59/2 (February 2011): 258–65; V. Kwok et al., "Learning New Color Names Produces Rapid Increase in Gray Matter in the Intact Adult Human Cortex," *Proceedings of the National Academy of Sciences* 108/16 (April 2011): 6686–88.

16. J. L. Mozolic et al., "A Cognitive Training Intervention Increases Resting Cerebral Blood Flow in Healthy Older Adults," *Frontiers in Human Neuroscience* 12/4 (March 2010): 16.

17. K. Alkadhi et al., "Neurobiological Consequences of Sleep Deprivation," *Current Neuro-pharmacology* 11/3 (May 2013): 231–49.

18. K. Karelina et al., "Oxytocin Mediates Social Neuroprotection After Cerebral Ischemia," *Stroke* 42/12 (December 2011): 3606–11.

19. Scott F. Owen et al., "Oxytocin Enhances Hippocampal Spike Transmission by Modulating Fast-Spiking Interneurons," *Nature* 500/7463 (August 2013): 458–62.

20. E. Luders et al., "The Unique Brain Anatomy of Meditation Practitioners: Alterations in Cortical Gyrification," *Frontiers in Human Neuroscience* 29/6 (February 2012): 34; doi: 10.3389/fnhum.2012.00034.

21. A. Masoumi et al., "1Alpha,25-Dihydroxyvitamin D3 Interacts with Curcuminoids to Stimulate Amyloid-Beta Clearance by Macrophages of Alzheimer's Disease Patients," *Journal of Alzheimer's Disease* 17/3 (2009): 703–17.

22. C. Zuccato and E. Cattaneo, "Brain-Derived Neurotrophic Factor in Neurodegenerative Diseases," *Nature Reviews Neurology* 5/6 (June 2009): 311–22.

23. F. Sofi et al., "Physical Activity and Risk of Cognitive Decline: A Meta-Analysis of Prospective Studies," *Journal of Internal Medicine* 269/1 (January 2011): 107–17.

24. "Exercise and Depression," Harvard Health Publications, http://www.health .harvard.edu/newsweek/Exercise-and-Depression-report-excerpt.htm.

25. M. H. Eskelinen et al., "Fat Intake at Midlife and Cognitive Impairment Later in Life: A Population-Based CAIDE Study," *International Journal of Geriatric Psychiatry* 23/7 (July 2008): 741–47; D. Benton et al., "The Influence of the Glycaemic Load of Breakfast on the Behaviour of Children in School," *Physiology and Behavior* 92/4 (November 2007): 717–24; T. S. Rao et al., "Understanding Nutrition, Depression and Mental Illness," *Indian Journal of Psychiatry* 50/2 (April 2008): 77–82.

26. E. Kassi and A. G. Papavassiliou, "Could Glucose Be a Proaging Factor?" *Journal of Cellular and Molecular Medicine* 12/4 (August 2008): 1194–98.

27. W. C. Willett et al., "Health Implications of Mediterranean Diets in Light of Contem-porary Knowledge, "1. Plant Foods and Dairy Products," *American Journal of Clinical Nutrition* 61/6 Suppl. (June 1995): 1407S–1415S; N. Tzima et al., "Mediterranean Diet and Insulin Sensitivity, Lipid Profile and Blood Pressure Levels, in Overweight and Obese People; The Attica Study," *Lipids in Health and Disease* 6 (September 2007): 22; A. Trichopoulou et al., "Adherence to a Mediterranean Diet and Survival in a Greek Population," *New England Journal of Medicine* 348/26 (June 2003): 2599–608.

28. N. Scarmeas et al., "Mediterranean Diet and Mild Cognitive Impairment," *Archives of Neurology* 66/2 (February 2009): 216–25.

29. S. T. Henderson et al., "Study of the Ketogenic Agent AC–1202 in Mild to Moderate Alzheimer's Disease: A Randomized, Double-Blind, Placebo-Controlled, Multicenter Trial," *Nutrition and Metabolism* (London) 6 (2009): 31.

30. R. Krikorian et al., "Blueberry Supplementation Improves Memory in Older Adults," *Journal of Agricultural and Food Chemistry* 58/7 (April 2010): 3996–4000; J. A. Joseph et al., "Reversals of Age-Related Declines in Neuronal Signal Transduction, Cognitive, and Motor Behavioral Deficits with Blueberry, Spinach, or Strawberry Dietary Supplementation," *Journal of Neuroscience* 19/18 (September 1999): 8114–21; D. H. Malin et al., "Short-Term Blueberry-Enriched Diet Prevents and Reverses Object Recognition Memory Loss in Aging Rats," *Nutrition* 27/3 (March 2011): 338–42.

31. J. A. Joseph et al., "Cellular and Behavioral Effects of Stilbene Resveratrol Analogues: Implications for Reducing the Deleterious Effects of Aging," *Journal of Agricultural and Food Chemistry* 56/22 (November 2008): 10544–51.

32. A. D. Smith et al., "Homocysteine-Lowering by B Vitamins Slows the Rate of Accelerated Brain Atrophy in Mild Cognitive Impairment: A Randomized Controlled Trial," *PLoS One* 5/9 (September 2010): e12244; doi: 10.1371/journal. pone.0012244.

Index

About the Author

Eva Selhub, M.D., is a lecturer in medicine at Harvard Medical School and a clinical associate of the Massachusetts General Hospital. She was medical director and senior physician at the Benson-Henry Institute for Mind/Body Medicine at the Massachusetts General Hospital for thirteen years. A trained internist and board certified in internal medicine, Dr. Selhub runs a private practice as a comprehensive medical specialist and transformation consultant. Visit her at www.drselhub.com.